The

SWISS SECRET

to Optimal Health

The
SWISS
SECRET
to Optimal Health

DR. RAU'S DIET FOR WHOLE BODY HEALING

Thomas Rau, M.D.
with Susan Wyler

BERKLEY BOOKS, NEW YORK

THE BERKLEY PUBLISHING GROUP
Published by the Penguin Group
Penguin Group (USA) Inc.
375 Hudson Street, New York, New York 10014, USA
Penguin Group (Canada), 90 Eglinton Avenue East, Suite 700, Toronto, Ontario M4P 2Y3, Canada
(a division of Pearson Penguin Canada Inc.)
Penguin Books Ltd., 80 Strand, London WC2R 0RL, England
Penguin Group Ireland, 25 St. Stephen's Green, Dublin 2, Ireland (a division of Penguin Books Ltd.)
Penguin Group (Australia), 250 Camberwell Road, Camberwell, Victoria 3124, Australia
(a division of Pearson Australia Group Pty. Ltd.)
Penguin Books India Pvt. Ltd., 11 Community Centre, Panchsheel Park, New Delhi—110 017, India
Penguin Group (NZ), 67 Apollo Drive, Mairangi Bay, Auckland 1311, New Zealand
(a division of Pearson New Zealand Ltd.)
Penguin Books (South Africa) (Pty.) Ltd., 24 Sturdee Avenue, Rosebank, Johannesburg 2196,
South Africa

Penguin Books Ltd., Registered Offices: 80 Strand, London WC2R 0RL, England

This book is an original publication of The Berkley Publishing Group.

Copyright © 2007 by Dr. Thomas Rau.
Text design by Tiffany Estreicher.
Illustrations on pages 4 and 109 by Pat Roberts.
Photographs on page 32 provided by the Paracelsus Clinic.

First edition: April 2007

Library of Congress Cataloging-in-Publication Data

Rau, Thomas, M.D.
    The Swiss secret to optimal health : Dr. Rau's diet for whole body healing / Thomas Rau, with Susan Wyler.
        p. cm.
    Includes index.
    ISBN 978-0-425-21393-3 (hardcover)
1. Health.   2. Nutrition.   3. Holistic medicine.   I. Wyler, Susan.   II. Paracelsus Klinic Lustmühle.   III. Title.

R733.R387 2007
613.2—dc22   2006101355

PRINTED IN THE UNITED STATES OF AMERICA

10   9   8   7   6   5   4   3   2

PUBLISHER'S NOTE: Every effort has been made to ensure that the information contained in this book is complete and
accurate. However, neither the publisher nor the author is engaged in rendering professional advice or services to the individual reader. The ideas, procedures, and suggestions contained in this book are not intended as a substitute for consulting with your physician. All matters regarding your health require medical supervision. Neither the author nor the
publisher shall be liable or responsible for any loss or damage allegedly arising from any information or suggestion in
this book.

The recipes contained in this book are to be followed exactly as written. The publisher is not responsible for your specific
health or allergy needs that may require medical supervision. The publisher is not responsible for any adverse reactions
to the recipes contained in this book.

While the author has made every effort to provide accurate telephone numbers and Internet addresses at the time of publication, neither the publisher nor the author assumes any responsibility for errors, or for changes that occur after publication. Further, publisher does not have any control over and does not assume any responsibility for author or third-party
websites or their content.

To my grandmother "Omama," who passed on to me her gift of intuitive knowing about people and who is still with me in spirit.

To my mother, who provided us with stability and a warm family life and always believed in the goodness of human beings.

To my father, who imbued me with a spirit of independence and taught me to follow my own thoughts.

To my wife, Elisabeth, who has supported my work through all these years with dedication, patience, and advice.

To my patients, from whom I have learned so much about life, love, courage in the face of fear, and the power of hope.

And to unconventional thinkers everywhere, who will continue to open new pathways to healing.

Thomas Rau, 2007

Contents

ACKNOWLEDGMENTS

This book, which is not only about a special diet and form of nutrition, but also about a very deep-healing form of biological medicine and a healthful way of living, came to life because I was asked again and again by many patients who came to the Paracelsus Clinic in Switzerland to record my recipes, so they could continue to follow our diet when they returned home. Many also wanted a greater understanding of Swiss biological medicine and of the benefits they were experiencing physically.

It is thanks to my partners in the United States, especially Margie and Michael Baldwin and the Marion Institute they founded, that I began to collect our recipes and write about the principles of Swiss biological medicine in language for the layman. It is thanks to Barbara Christian, director of the Paracelsus Biological Medicine Network, who organized me, stood behind me, and pushed me, that I finally began to write my work down. Barbara also brought me together with chef and cookbook author Kathi Long, who has since moved to join us at Paracelsus and is now chef at our clinic restaurant.

Without Kathi, I wouldn't have met my co-author, Susan Wyler, who made it possible to complete this book and who brought my theories and my work into a language that is understandable for everyone. Over and over, Susan questioned me and insisted I explain everything. Thank you, dear Susan, for all your endless work and dedication to my work. Without you this book would have never been born.

Thanks also to my excellent publisher, Berkley Books, and to our discerning editor, Denise Silvestro, who understood my work from the beginning and was so instrumental in creating this beautiful book.

Learning biological medicine is a lifelong path filled with dedication, respect of nature, and love. It requires intuitive learning and association with many teachers and philosophers. There were several on my path:

My friend and former teacher, Dr. Konrad Werthmann, who researched food allergies for more than 30 years and who taught me about his professor, Dr. Günther Enderlein. He was also the first to show me the correlation between hidden food allergies and chronic diseases. Konrad, I learned a lot from you!

Mr. Jürg Binz, who introduced me to the Sanum Remedies. In 1990, we decided to take over the Paracelsus Clinic together, which gave me the opportunity to treat my patients with widespread Paracelsus Biological Medicine remedies, milieu therapy, and diet.

Thanks to all my friends and teachers in Germany and Austria, including Professor Arno Rost and Dr. Jochen Gleditsch, as well as my colleagues in the United States, including Dr. James Odell.

Many thanks also to my supporters in the United States, especially Mr. Rainer Kehlbeck, owner of the Sanum Kehlbeck company, and their U.S. representatives, Mrs. Christyne Jackson and Colonel Felix Müller of Pleomorphic Product Sales, Inc.

All my work, my many seminars, my presence in our cooperative clinics all over the world, and my writing would not be possible without my Paracelsus Clinic Lustmühle, Switzerland, where my colleagues and partners have supported me for so many years in their daily work. Special thanks to my friend and partner from the beginning, Dr. Victor von Toenges, M.D., from whom I learned anthroposophical medicine. He imbues the clinic with sense of continuity and humanity.

Thanks to Irene Guler, whose vegetarian alkaline cooking in our hotel and clinic created such a demand for our recipes.

I also want to thank Mr. Ronald Sutter, our "information officer" and chief secretary of the "Verlag der Paracelsus Klinik" (publications and editions) for all his detail work, and my chief secretary, Mrs. Rosemary Lutz, who organizes me so well here in Switzerland.

—Dr. Thomas M. Rau, M.D.

There are many people who were involved in the production of this book whom I'd like to thank:

Chef Kathi Long, who first thought Dr. Rau's nutrition should be codified and recorded in a book.

Barbara Christian, director of the Paracelsus Biological Medicine Network, who refers patients every day and who generously introduced me to the seminars in this country and helped me understand biological medicine at the outset.

Michael and Margie Baldwin, whose support of the Biological Medicine Network has been invaluable.

My excellent editor, Denise Silvestro, who understood from the outset what this book is all about; and assistant editor Katie Day, for all her attention to detail.

Christian and Irene Guler, whose hospitality in Switzerland helped make this book possible.

All those who helped me with the recipes: Kathi Long, Irene Guler, Peggy Fallon, and Ken Charney.

Elisabeth Rau, whose keen eye and knowledge of both cooking and nutrition helped vet all the recipes in the book.

And, of course, special thanks to Dr. Thomas Rau, whose life's work offers hope to so many.

—Susan Wyler

The evolution of medicine moves slowly. *The Swiss Secret to Optimal Health* by Dr. Thomas Rau takes medicine to the next level of evolution. Over 125 million Americans suffer from chronic disease for which there is little more than remedial treatment to suppress symptoms with drugs that interfere with or block normal physiology.

Dr. Rau presents a new vision of healing that addresses chronic disease in a revolutionary way. He practices medicine in the tradition of William Osler, one of the founding fathers of modern medicine, who said, "It is more important to treat the patient that has the disease, than the disease that the patient has."

Swiss biological medicine is a way of seeing health and disease that does exactly that. The principles of this new medicine shift dramatically from trying to find the name of the disease (or diseases) that a person has to a deep understanding of the underlying causes of disease (such as toxins, infections, allergens, stress), and ways to remove those causes and then help support and encourage the body's natural healing systems. The disease, then, takes care of itself. This is what America needs in a spiraling epidemic of chronic disease and escalating health care costs.

The tools and methods of biological medicine focus on supporting the body's normal powers of regeneration, regulation, and healing. This perspective utilizes emerging scientific research on systems biology and medicine and nutrition, and offers a truly new solution to people who suffer from chronic health conditions. Rather than focus on treating a specific disease and using medication (as conventional doctors are trained to do), Dr. Rau and the other proponents of biological medicine use cutting-edge technologies to assess and diagnose underlying imbalances, and novel treatments to address the underlying causes of disease such as toxicity, inflammation, and immune and digestive imbalances.

This type of medicine gets to the root of illness. *The Swiss Secret to Optimal Health* will help you do this in three critical ways. First, by helping you detoxify from living in a toxic world. Second, by changing our acidic, poor quality, processed food, high-sugar, high-meat and high-protein diet to a more alkaline and healing diet of whole foods, fresh vegetables, fruits, nuts and seeds, whole grains, legumes, and small amounts of lean animal protein. And lastly, by helping us correct digestive systems damaged by a poor diet and by the overuse of antibiotics, hormones, anti-inflammatory medicines, and stress. These are the pillars of Dr. Rau's Swiss Secret. For those suffering from chronic illness, or those who just want to feel how good they can feel, I recommend trying Dr. Rau's Swiss Detox Diet.

There has been a remarkable parallel evolution of medicine in America. It is called functional medicine (www.functionalmedicine.org) and applies nearly identical principles to address the underlying causes of disease, and to support and encourage the body's own healing mechanisms. I have been a practitioner and teacher of this new medicine for over 10 years.

Biological medicine and functional medicine are the practical applications of this remarkable new evolutionary leap and provide a way for the average person to take control of his or her health and escape from the prison of chronic illness and poor quality of life. The refrain I often hear from my patients who apply these principles (as you can do by following *The Swiss Secret to Optimal Health*) is, "I didn't know how bad I was feeling until I started feeling so good!"

Mark Hyman, M.D.
Lenox, MA
January 4, 2007

Exploring the Puzzle

THOMAS RAU, M.D.

Swiss biological medicine has been an important part of my life for more than 25 years. My involvement with it began well after I had trained and specialized as a traditional medical doctor, and my commitment to it strengthens with each passing year. This holistic medical approach appeals to different parts of me: my altruistic medical instincts, because I see how effectively it helps my patients in a way orthodox medicine does not; my emotions, because in many ways a biological practitioner relates to his or her patient in an empathic way traditional medicine has until very recently discouraged; and especially my intellect, because each patient, according to this scheme, is approached as a unique individual, whose many symptoms represent a puzzle that must be solved.

The most basic tenet of the broad-based holistic medicine we practice at my clinic in Switzerland, the Paracelsus Clinic Lustmühle, is that we treat individuals, not just symptoms or diseases. If you've explored alternative medicine, you may have heard this before, but it is integral to our approach. Two people might come to me, both suffering from migraine headaches or a persistent rash, and I would know that in order to help them, I must assume that the basis of the same symptom in each patient might well be completely different. The same applies to the root causes of chronic and even serious inflammatory and degenerative diseases.

This model of the patient as a unique organism who needs individualized treatments makes perfect sense once you learn a little about the theory of Swiss biological medicine. I like to compare it to a project I had in school when I was quite young.

Like many boys at that time, I was required to take shop along with all my academic subjects. One day in woodworking class, as we were being taught how to use a band saw, we were given a relatively simple assignment. We were each handed a photograph of our hometown, Teufen, which we were instructed to paste onto a flat board. The task was to cut out a dozen pieces from the board to make a jigsaw puzzle. How does this relate to biological medicine and the uniqueness of each patient?

Well, the whole class began with exactly the same picture. But each of us ended up with a different puzzle. Not a single piece from one boy's puzzle fit together with any other piece in the entire room. And that is how we look at the biological makeup of each person.

The differences among people arise from their genetic makeup, their life experiences, what toxins they have inadvertently been exposed to, what medicines they have taken, and what they choose to eat on a daily basis, among other things. One person lives in the city; another in the country. One swims every day; another leads a sedentary life. It all adds up, and all the patterns are different.

Of course, if you come to our clinic in Switzerland, we solve the puzzle for you. But I wrote this book in the hope that intelligent people everywhere who wish to be responsible for their health and overall well-being and who want to feel better will attempt to solve the puzzle for themselves so that they, too, can benefit from our biological medicine. To help you understand *why* we suggest the particular balance of foods and what's behind the dos and don'ts detailed in Dr. Rau's Way—my two-step nutritional program—I've explained the theory in separate chapters.

Whether you read the more scientific chapters that explain the theory behind what we prescribe or you simply flip to the nutrition chapters and cook the recipes at the back of the book to follow my diet, in these pages you will find something that adds significantly to your physical well-being. Help is here; how far you take it is up to you.

While each patient is an individual and requires a unique plan of treatment, our basic nutrition plan is excellent for almost all people and for a very wide range of medical problems. As they say, preventative medicine is the best medicine, and Swiss biological medicine believes this maxim above all. It's just that our preventative medicine is a little different: It's a rich nutritional plan unlike any other you have ever tried. And while it works exceedingly well preemptively, it also has tremendous palliative and healing power.

The first stage of Dr. Rau's Way, the Swiss Detox Diet, is for almost everyone. It produces striking results in a very short period of time: just three short weeks. After that, when you move on to my Maintenance Diet for Life, it is up to you—with our careful guidance—to unlock your own secrets and determine the very best way for you to eat for your individual needs and to support your health.

For the average person who is in reasonably good health, our nutritional plan offers an excellent tonic for warding off both illness and what we too often accept as the inevitable diminishing of our physical and mental powers as we age. I would be willing to bet that at least 95 percent of average people, even those who *think* they have no physical problems, will benefit enormously from this program. For everything about Dr. Rau's Way is designed to support and enhance the natural vitality and healing potential of the human being.

Many healthy people come to me hoping simply to feel better as they age or to try to avoid a genetic propensity like heart disease or cancer that they know runs in their family. Other people come to me for the serious chronic inflammatory, degenerative, and autoimmune diseases I specialized in as a young man: severe allergies, rheumatoid arthritis, digestive problems, persistent skin rashes. I enjoy welcoming these patients especially, because I have witnessed our type of biological medicine to be so effective at dealing with these systemic illnesses. We also see many cancer patients as well as people suffering from chronic fatigue syndrome, fibromyalgia, obesity, and the type 2 diabetes that often accompanies this condition. And then there are the patients with psychological or mental problems, such as depression, ADDS (attention deficient and distress syndrome), autism, and hyperactivity, especially in children. We see all these maladies as inextricably connected to the patient's physical condition as well; and here, too, I believe our diet confers tremendous benefits.

The reason I am so pleased to offer this book to you is that unlike many other health systems, with Swiss biological medicine, neither the doctor nor the patient is alone. The effectiveness of the treatment is based on a pact between the two: a sensitive, open-minded, trained professional and a proactive patient who is willing—and eager—to participate in his or her cure.

By cure, I don't mean just swallowing a pill, but easing or removing the symptoms by eradicating the underlying reasons for whatever the ailment happens to be—whether an illness with an important name or a constellation of vague symptoms that interfere with your full enjoyment of your family, your profession, and your life.

Since the basis of all my medicine is nutrition, the effectiveness of Swiss biological medicine can, in large part at least, begin at home. The goal of this book is to offer you not just a diet, but enough information so that you can understand where many of your symptoms are coming from. Of course, this is no way prevents you from consulting a traditional medical doctor for any illness you have already or think you may be developing. But I am confident that if you follow Dr. Rau's Way, it will over time offer you a level of vitality and wellness you will find nowhere else.

A NOTE FROM
CO-AUTHOR SUSAN WYLER

If truth be told, I began work on this book with only mild interest and no small degree of skepticism. As both author and editor, my professional life has been consumed with writing about high-end food, and my personal life with the enjoyment of said food. Diets have held no interest for me. During graduate studies, I had some science training and a laboratory job in a most distinguished research facility. That very rational point of view suits my temperament to this day, which means that when I began this project, I approached what I viewed as "alternative medicine" with a questioning, if not cynical, eye. Needless to say, I have become a complete convert, and the transformation arose from firsthand experience.

I had never explored any kind of alternative medicine. I like all my doctors. Despite metabolic problems common to many postmenopausal women and the gradual decline that I thought invariably came with age, I considered myself healthy. I took Synthroid for a slow thyroid and had a problem with cholesterol—both my parents had bypass operations—and, oh, yes, my doctor was threatening me with blood pressure medication; but still, I thought of myself as healthy. I had seasonal allergies. In fact, for a couple of years, I called myself the queen of Allegra, but all my friends suffered as well. I considered it part of the human condition—at least for that segment of the population that was fortunate enough to spend time in the countryside.

The food I ate every day was extremely delicious and, I thought, wholesome. Weight was never a big problem, but if I became a bit chunky through sloth and wanted to lose weight, I simply cut out bread and wine and ate less for a few weeks. I thought people were hypochondriacs when they said they were allergic to different foods.

And so it was in this callow state of mind that I met Dr. Rau for the first time at a biological medicine conference in Massachusetts. In preparation for writing this book, I put myself on his Swiss Detox Diet. While one might lose weight easily on this plan, the intention, I was told, was to improve your health by nourishing the basic internal environment of your body. Whatever, I thought. It has nothing to do with me. The real question I worried about was, can you stay on this diet for three weeks and not get depressed for lack of culinary pleasure?

In fact, Dr. Rau's diet was very satisfying; but much more importantly, it had such an immediate and dramatic impact upon how I felt and upon my measurable health that it startled me and surprised even my internist. I am still on the diet, and my general health continues to improve—both in ways important to Swiss biological medicine and in ways my traditional doctors measure each time I see them. Here is what happened to me.

After only three or four days on the diet, I noticed a change in my gut. It felt distinctly lighter, clearer; there were no rumblings and grumblings. My intestinal tract had been bloated or irritated in some way, and I didn't even realize it until the sensations disappeared. Then, after 10 days, my energy, which had been very much on the low side, noticeably soared. Best of all, it remained constant all day. I was amazed at how rejuvenated I felt. Friends started complimenting me on how well I looked.

This improvement continued over time. I've never needed more than seven hours' sleep. But whether I got a lot or a little, my entire life I was never able to get out of bed in the morning. I read that there were two kinds of people: those whose endocrine systems were up and going when they woke up and those whose system took about an hour to rev up. Certainly, I was one of the latter, only mine took more like an hour and a half. Mornings were excruciating.

No more. Now, whether I get my usual seven hours of sleep or under deadline only four or five, I wake up bright and energetic, ready to go even before my first—and last—cup of coffee of the day. For what it's worth, I lost 12 pounds the first two months, a lot for a woman my size, and that was while packing away more food than I thought I could possibly eat. What's more, I have kept it off.

I feel consistently more alert and able to focus clearly; my memory, which seemed dodgy for a while, has improved greatly; and I feel calmer. Bouts of mild depression, which occasionally visited on and off for years, have disappeared. My overall anxiety level is greatly lessened. My energy level and stamina are tremendous. And, as Dr. Rau would have predicted, my seasonal allergies have disappeared.

My blood pressure has dropped 15 to 20 points. While without any drugs my cholesterol remains higher than recommended, my good cholesterol continues to rise and the bad to fall, so that my ratio is extremely good; it gets better each time I am tested. By biological medicine standards, my blood has improved markedly during this time.

What has thrilled me most is the improvement in my thyroid condition. While I complained about symptoms for years, I always tested low normal rather than pathological, so I was never prescribed any medication. Only when an unsightly goiter finally developed around my neck was my condition acknowledged and treated with Synthroid.

"Will it go away now that I'm taking medication?" I asked my endocrinologist hopefully, eyeing the bulging tire around my lower neck. "No," she replied, "but it won't get any bigger." It didn't, nor did it get any smaller . . . for seven years.

After eight months on the diet, I looked in the mirror one day and could have sworn my neck was thinner. Must be my imagination, I thought. A few days later it was unmistakable and within a month and a half, the goiter simply melted away. Best of all, my thyroid function as measured by standard hormone tests improved 25 percent, most unusual during a time in life when metabolic processes tend to slow down, if anything. How nice to have to reduce your medication.

And the food, you ask? Now when my friends come over to dinner, they ask ahead of time, "Will you make me a Dr. Rau salad, please?" That's because they are so attractive and delicious, and they make you feel so good. The diet is not strictly vegetarian, but fresh fruits, whole grains, and especially vegetables are important, and that's the new part for me. I've discovered how delicious organic vegetables taste—raw, steamed, and lightly cooked—and I realize that this nutritional plan fits in perfectly with the contemporary fine-food movement: It advocates the best, purest food, simply prepared, beautifully served, and offered up with love. I sincerely hope you'll give Dr. Rau's Way a chance to improve your health as well as enhance how you look and feel every day.

CHAPTER ONE

Understanding Swiss Biological Medicine

YOUR NATURAL PATH TO HEALTH

Since you've opened this book, there's a good chance you've been let down in some way by orthodox medicine and you are searching for help. Perhaps you're one of the millions of people suffering from chronic pain, relentless headaches, sinus infections, chronic fatigue syndrome, unexplained listlessness, allergies, or an inability to focus. You may have received no helpful diagnosis, or you may have received a life-challenging diagnosis, such as multiple sclerosis (MS), cancer, or rheumatoid arthritis. You may be afflicted with a subclinical illness, feel old before your time, or want to ward off a hereditary tendency that runs in your family. Or you may simply wish to look and feel as good as you can for as long as possible.

You've already taken the most important step: you've opened your mind to possibilities. As I tell all my patients, *healing requires a commitment to change.* If you're not well, you must turn around and face in another direction.

Swiss biological medicine offers a comprehensive program of natural healing that approaches illness from a completely different point of view from traditional orthodox medicine. Rather than seeing health primarily as a war that pits your body against outside invaders (e.g., germs, viruses, and other pathogens), we believe the healthy body is in balance with itself and with the physical world in which it exists. Illness arises from within when that equilibrium is breached. This may sound poetic, but the balance we speak of is more literal than figurative.

While external factors, of course, have an effect on people, many bacteria and viruses—and even cancer cells—are floating about all the time and arising within our bodies every day. A well-tuned immune system knocks them out. Given any particular illness, only a certain proportion of the population gets sick, no matter what its exposure. And of those who do get sick, only a certain proportion dies. The variability lies within the individual. *Good health can only prevail within a well-regulated body.*

At the heart of a body in balance is proper nutrition. No matter what other "bag of tricks" I may have at hand as a medical doctor, it is your personal day-to-day dietary habits that will ultimately determine your physical quality of life. To promote the best health possible and to provide the platform for other biological medicine treatments, this book introduces Dr. Rau's Way, a two-step diet that forms the bedrock of my medical beliefs. In a very broad way, it is a diet low in animal protein and rich in vegetables, whole grains, and fruits. These foods provide a large amount of vitamins, minerals, trace elements, essential amino acids, and highly unsaturated fatty acids. But the diet's power to significantly affect your health lies in the details that boost your life energy, which are laid out in the chapters that follow.

The number of diet books that list what you can and cannot eat based on purely arbitrary standards and bogus assumptions astonishes me. Read half a dozen acid/alkaline diet books, and you'll find six different lists of which vegetables you may and may not eat. In fact, science is not arbitrary at all. For every food I prohibit or promote, there is a reason that is the case, and that reason is based on the precepts of Swiss biological medicine. To completely understand the diet, you should first understand the medicine. *To act differently, you must first think differently.*

If science bores you, you can at any time simply skip to the chapters that spell out what you can and cannot eat and how the stages of the diet progress. For anyone who wants only the nuts and bolts of the diet, at the back of the book you'll find more than 100 easy-to-follow recipes that conform to my dietary principles. However, I believe firmly that knowledge is power. It's much easier to follow any rule when you understand *why* it has been established. That said, I hope you will read on to gain a basic understanding of Swiss biological medicine—our theory and our treatments—and why this natural form of healing works so effectively.

Lightening Your Toxic Load

To promote vitality and to enjoy the ability to grow and heal itself, a person's internal environment must exhibit two fundamental properties: the fluids that flow through the body—blood and lymphatic fluids—as well as the interstitial fluids that surround every cell must be slightly alkaline in order to counter the acidity that is a natural by-product of cell metabolism; and the intestinal flora (bacteria) must be intact and healthy. (There are many reasons for this, which I will explain in detail a later on.)

Without such "fertile soil," illness arises sooner or later when the balance tips and the person loses his or her regulatory powers, usually as a result of not one but several insults to the system. These "forces of evil," if you will, we call "toxic load." Many physical and mental problems, as well as inadvertent exposure to toxic materials in the environment, can put a body out of balance. The goal of Swiss biological medicine is to remove those toxins and get the body back in balance to allow your natural defenses and vitality to thrive.

My favorite metaphor for the body in relation to its health is that of a big oil barrel. When you are born, your body is fresh, pure, and strong. It's a new, empty barrel that offers plenty of storage. Which is good, because life is messy, and you accumulate a lot of "junk." You are exposed to germs, toxins, and pollutants. You may eat the "wrong" foods, undergo undue stress, or become contaminated with heavy metals through seafood

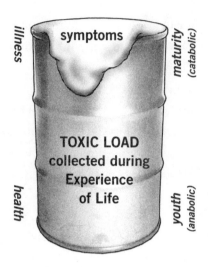

or dental fillings. All these detrimental intrusions can interfere with the flow of energy within your body and slow down your immune system and vital metabolic processes.

But when you are young and your up-building, or anabolic, forces are still extremely strong, all of this toxic load is dumped into the empty space in the barrel, leaving you vital and seemingly healthy . . . at least for a while. Over time, however, toxins, poisons, trans fats and excess proteins, injuries, abuse of alcohol and tobacco, residues from stress and genetic weaknesses, overeating, not getting enough exercise or sleep, being exposed to air pollution, and taking drugs—recreational and pharmaceutical (especially antibiotics)—add to the toxic load in the barrel and it begins to fill up.

Yet even if the barrel is three quarters full, you may still insist you are absolutely fine. After all, your body compensates as much as it possibly can before giving in. Or you may attribute symptoms like fatigue, lack of concentration, forgetfulness, lack of sexual drive, and depression to other factors entirely: age, menopause, working too hard, something you ate or didn't eat.

Eventually, the poisons reach the top and the barrel overflows. Essentially your body loses its battle against all the physical insults and tips out of balance and you fall ill. Thus, a disease usually has not just one but multiple causes. That's why, as practitioners of biological medicine, we treat the entire individual and not just a single symptom.

To effect our cures, Swiss biological medicine incorporates an integrated holistic approach, employing alternative treatments—some of which have proven their effectiveness over hundreds, and sometimes thousands, of years—along with isopathic and homeopathic remedies and other procedures that rely on state-of-the-art contemporary equipment and biochemistry. These techniques are complemented with the most up-to-date diagnostic procedures and technical advances in traditional modern medicine. Despite all the science and wide array of treatments, however, at the heart of this medicine lies the most important variable over which only the patient ultimately has control: nutrition.

What you eat is the single most important contribution you can make to your own health. Nutrition is the vital key that determines the condition of the body's internal environment. That is why I developed my easy-to-follow dietary program: Dr. Rau's Way.

Who Benefits and Why

This type of holistic medicine is particularly effective at dealing with chronic inflammatory and degenerative diseases, including allergies, arthritis, atherosclerosis, arterial sclerosis, congestive heart disease, MS, lupus, asthma, acid reflux, fibromyalgia, chronic infections, and cancer. We also have very good results with mental diseases, such as depression, bipolar disorder, hyperactivity, and autism.

There is also another group of extremely common diseases that are greatly benefited by Swiss biological medicine. These conditions include all the "deposit" diseases, pathological problems that arise when the body deals with materials it cannot process by storing them in the blood, interstitial spaces, or even within the tissues. Examples are obesity, coronary heart disease, hypertension, type 2 diabetes, and microcirculation deficiency.

As anyone who has suffered from a major illness or watched a loved one struggle with a degenerative ailment knows, Western medicine does not have many answers to chronic disease. When it comes to systemic diseases, traditional (allopathic) doctors tend to treat symptoms randomly rather than to address the root causes of the disease, which in many cases are still not well understood and which vary from patient to patient.

In fact, as I stated earlier, there are usually multiple causes that give rise to an illness. The reason Swiss biological medicine is so effective at alleviating, and in many cases curing, this range of ills is that it approaches health and disease in a completely different way from conventional medicine, marshaling the body's natural defenses to effectively bring about its own healing rather than trying to knock out an individual symptom, such as a fever or rash, with a pharmaceutical drug.

Practitioners of biological medicine see such symptoms not as a flaw, but as a physical manifestation of the body's attempt to put itself back in balance. So these symptoms give us clues as to what the real problem or problems are. And when we address those underlying difficulties, which invariably relate to the patient's internal environment, the symptoms disappear by themselves.

Some Limitations of Traditional Medicine

Pharmaceutical drugs, on the other hand, not only do not cure the underlying cause of a disease, they damage the body in the process of trying. For every action, there is a reaction, and every pharmaceutical drug has some side effect, whether it's destroying good intestinal bacteria, as in the case of antibiotics, or causing excessive stomach bleeding, as in the case of too much aspirin and other anti-inflammatory drugs.

Overuse of acetaminophen in the presence of alcohol has resulted in serious liver damage. Some of us are old enough to remember the tragedy of thalidomide, which resulted in tens of thousands of babies being born with no arms, their hands attached at the shoulders. Often we read how a drug touted in banner headlines as the ultimate panacea for a particular ailment has no effect whatsoever, despite claims to the contrary that have been popularly accepted for many, many years.

Most shocking, according to the article "New Drugs Hit the Market, but Promised Trials Go Undone," (Gardiner Harris, *New York Times* online, March 4, 2006), which examined lax oversight of pharmaceutical drugs by the U.S. Food and Drug Administration (FDA), is that the real physical effects of many drugs—both positive and negative—are rarely proven in scientific trials. Because of problems involved in conducting so-called double-blind studies, only one in five drugs used to fight cancer has been statistically proven to extend the length of patients' lives. That's because once a drug shows any promise, doctors are reluctant to withhold it to complete their statistical studies. In addition, damaging side effects of these drugs are often underreported. So the actual practice is often just trial and error. What we are led to believe is 100 percent cut-and-dried science is, at heart, equal parts art and intuition.

When studies are conducted, they are often extremely fallible, and the conclusions are easily manipulated. Tests that seem so technical are, in fact, easy to skew, often unconsciously, owing to the bias of the testers, the group sampled, the structure of the study, the variables considered, the wording of questionnaires, and the interpretation of the statistics.

My thinking is that practitioners of Western medicine need to understand that the human being is so complex it cannot be measured with one variable. The double-blind study often fails because it doesn't take into account the complexity of human functions; by its very nature it is structured to assume that each individual is the same.

Practitioners of Swiss biological medicine treat each person as a unique individual with his or her own medical needs and tendencies. Based on a person's particular DNA, constitutional makeup, and personal life experiences—both physical and psychological—we tailor the treatment to fit the patient. Once you are familiar with the Swiss biological way, I am confident you will look at your health from a completely different vantage point.

Scientific Theory Behind the Medicine

What may surprise new patients is the model of health and illness that Swiss biological medicine posits. It is a very different one from that of the orthodox Western medical establishment, or what I call "school medicine," whose description of illness is based on the work of Louis Pasteur. Basically, Pasteur's theory, developed in the 1880s, views all infectious illness as a result of pathogens (i.e., germs) that come from outside the body and invade an otherwise passive environment (the body), thus causing symptoms and suffering.

Integrated biological medicine as practiced at the Paracelsus Clinic in Switzerland embraces many traditions and practices, but theoretically it is based on a dynamic model of the body's internal environment. We see a constant up-building and degrading, an ebb and flow taking place, with health being determined by a regulated body that is in balance. Disease occurs when the internal environment is degraded by one or more disturbances: poor diet, heavy metal contamination, electromagnetic contamination, toxic pollution, undetected dental infections, chronic psychological stress, etc. By modifying your internal environment—especially the intestinal flora, the blood, the lymph system, and the interstitial fluids—and by bringing the body back into balance, you can restore and maintain good health.

This *pleomorphic* view of health was developed in the 1920s by a medical doctor named Günther Enderlein. Using high-powered microscopes available to him, which were not developed in Pasteur's day, Enderlein identified tiny microorganisms in the blood. Strangely, these tiny "symbionts," as he called them, could not be destroyed, even by extremely high heat. He posited that these minute creatures, consisting of bits of protein, live in helpful symbiosis with the body when the body's metabolism and biochemistry are in balance, much like the good bacteria in the intestinal tract. We believe these symbionts in their benign state are important to the vitality of all cells, acting as catalysts in the formation of many cellular functions and vital to the up-building of the essential intestinal flora.

Just as we need the bacteria in our gastrointestinal system, we need these microorganisms so we can function smoothly. In fact, if we don't see enough symbionts when we examine a person's blood, we consider the patient run-down and lacking internal vitality. We know we must build them up.

When wrong nutrition upsets the body's optimum balance, it shifts the natural alkalinity of your internal landscape, which supports good health, into an acidic state. This balance is quite tangible; it is reflected in the pH value (acidity level) of your blood, saliva, and interstitial fluids. When the balance tips, many physical changes occur. These include a thickening of the blood and lymph fluid, similar to the curdling of milk by the acid of lemon juice or vinegar; damage to the intestinal flora; and a change in the behavior of the symbionts and intestinal bacteria.

Under acidic conditions, those previously benign symbionts become agitated and corrupted into pathogens, mutating first into harmful bacteria, then to fungi or, if there are electromagnetic or toxic blockages in the body, to viruses. We call these different levels of energy *valences*. Like the electrons around an atom, it takes a certain amount of disturbance to energize these microorganisms enough so they jump to the next level.

Luckily, by regulating and rebalancing the body's internal environment—converting it back to an alkaline state, purging toxic loads, avoiding food allergies, and nurturing the immune system—health can be restored, because with the "soil" properly fertilized, those pathogens can be coaxed back into their benign form.

If you're like many, you may find this theory confusing at first. It is alien to what we were all taught growing up, and it remains controversial. But you can easily understand it in a conceptual way. As I've said, rather than seeing illness as an invasion from the outside (so that you would "catch" the flu), which is the approach traditional medicine takes, Swiss biological medicine believes our cells are in a constant state of flux and

THE BODY'S BALANCING ACT

Throughout your life, your health is like a ride on a seesaw; there is a constant interaction—and sometimes battle—between up-building and downgrading forces. All human bodies are in a permanent state of change. In seven years, not a single cell in your body will be the same as it is today. New cells constantly grow; old cells die and decay. It is part of the natural life cycle. Babies and young children have an intensive strength; their up-building, or anabolic, forces are powerful. Old people have an overload of so-called degenerative forces; the cells of their organs slow down and can no longer regenerate well.

When a young individual is subjected to an overload of degenerative forces, he or she will develop degenerative diseases early in life, such as

- Arterial blockages and coronary heart disease
- Brain or neurological deficiencies
- Degenerative joint diseases
- Macular degeneration

To turn around this increased tendency toward degeneration to a more anabolic, or up-building, direction, Swiss biological medicine tries to fortify all the organs in the body that by their nature have strong regenerative forces: the intestinal flora, the small intestines, the liver, the red and white blood cells, the bone marrow, and—most importantly—the parasympathetic, unconscious nervous system, which affects the heart rate, blood pressure, and ability to digest food, absorb nutrients, and excrete waste. This is done by alkalizing all the tissues in the body, which supports the up-building process, and by providing hormone-stimulating herbs and therapies.

that illness arises from within the individual when internal conditions weaken and illness overcomes our natural robust vitality. There is constant play between up-building and downgrading on a molecular level, and our entire medical program is aimed at regulating the body so that it is in a healthy balance and your immune system is as strong as it can be.

Our success at the Paracelsus Clinic comes from our approach to medicine, which, as noted, is devoted to treating the individual patient, not just vanquishing outward symptoms of a broad-based disease. By uncovering and removing the particular toxic load carried by each person and by nurturing him or her in every way possible, the body is given the support it needs to express itself in its naturally healthy form.

And where there can be no ultimate victory, we assist our patients in living each day with comfort and dignity as long as is possible. Helping is not always measured by healing. Sometimes it means providing a better quality of life. This is nearly always possible with Swiss biological medicine, even in progressed cancer cases.

Swiss biological medicine, framed within this model, works. And it works for a wide range of systemic, autoimmune, inflammatory, and degenerative diseases. It works for everything from allergies to cancer. I have seen this in the successes with our patients we have been treating for over 40 years. (The Paracelsus Clinic was founded in 1956; I have been medical director since 1992.)

To me, this model of medicine is extremely logical. That's why we call it bio*logical* medicine. But if it feels a little strange to you, think about all the theories of the physical world. Newtonian physics, which explains gravity, acceleration, and friction on a day-to-day level, worked perfectly well in describing the laws of motion for 250 years. In fact, it is still useful for explaining many of the physical events we witness every day.

When new ways of measuring mass and energy came into being, however, Newtonian physics took a backseat to Albert Einstein's revolutionary theories, which described the universe breathtakingly accurately on an atomic level, explaining the primal relationship between matter and energy—indeed positing that they are two forms of the same element. Then along came quantum theory, which works even better than Einstein's principles at describing certain behaviors of subatomic particles. Today, while scientists search for the perfect unified theory that will account for everything in the universe, they use both Einstein's theory of relativity and quantum mechanics because the two together are able to describe most of what we know about the physical world.

So it is with traditional (allopathic) medicine and the isopathic model developed by Enderlein. They sometimes work together. If my patient has a malignant tumor, I must turn to allopathic medicine and surgically remove it; and then I may have to treat the patient with some chemotherapy and perhaps radiation, because if the tumor is not stopped, I cannot do my real work: to bring about a lasting cure based on removing hidden toxic load and regulating the patient's internal environment. I need to buy time, to find out what is wrong at the deepest level, what caused that tumor to arise in the first place. Only then can we correct it. We treat not only the cancer but, more importantly, the causes behind it. I believe it is because of this that I have observed patients at Paracelsus Clinic experience less recurrence of cancer after undergoing Swiss biological medicine treatment.

Thus, especially with cancer, I use traditional procedures and drugs when absolutely necessary to buy time. However, the basis of all healing and the maintenance of good health belong to biological medicine.

My Path to Biological Medicine

I am very familiar with the orthodox American Medical Association (AMA) school of medicine because I am a medical doctor, an M.D., licensed to practice in both Switzerland and the United States. Early on in my career as an orthodox doctor with a specialty practice in rheumatology, I learned that traditional Western medicine was not particularly adept at dealing with chronic degenerative diseases. These include most of the noninfectious physical problems we all suffer from, especially as we age:

allergies, arthritis, arterial sclerosis, and other autoimmune and inflammatory diseases.

But it was only after many years of treating patients in a thriving practice that I began to question what I had been taught. I became discouraged because, while at first I successfully eliminated people's symptoms, my patients' problems persisted, and they had to keep coming back for regular treatments. In fact, as the years passed, most got worse and needed stronger medication or more frequent shots to suppress their symptoms. Eventually, it became clear to me that while I was a master of making symptoms disappear, the real cause of the illness was left untouched.

Once in a while, though, a patient would experience a so-called "spontaneous cure." I would notice that a regular patient would come in exhibiting more robust energy, acting alert and energetic, and reporting that her symptoms had subsided. "What did you do differently during these past few months?" I always asked.

"Well," one might say, "a friend recommended a book that says you should not eat any dairy or wheat, and I decided to try it." Another patient might have followed a different plan—perhaps a course of Chinese herbal teas—and also had good results. One patient I had been seeing for almost a decade became a strict vegetarian. Over a period of time, her health improved markedly, and after six months, her rheumatoid arthritis had nearly disappeared.

I listened closely—I am a very good listener—and over time, after a great deal of reading, studying, and doing research, it became clear to me there were alternative ways to practice medicine that were often more fundamentally effective than the course I had been pursuing. Perhaps what was viewed as a spontaneous cure was simply a kind of healing that marched to a different drummer.

Without discarding all the good I learned in school, I thought, Why are we so restricted in our choices? Why do we have to practice medicine along one narrow pathway and ignore all the other forms of healing so readily available to us? I read voraciously, learning alternative theories about illness and infection. I studied closely the work of Enderlein and of another doctor, H. H. Reckeweg, who united allopathic and isopathic medicine with his homeopathic remedies. I found myself in agreement with them about the dynamic concept of up-building and degeneration in the body and about the importance of regulating the system and removing blockages to good health.

It made sense to me that much of good health consists of coming into a kind of physical balance, or regulation. Much as you fine-tune a mechanical clock to keep the many cogs in the mechanism in sync or adjust the balance of a metronome to keep perfect time, each person's body needs help finding its own rhythm, its own balance. Slowly, I began to see that there was a much larger world of healing at my fingertips. There were many techniques that could help a patient, even if they were not officially sanctioned by mainstream medical societies. After all, many of these treatments—homeopathy, acupuncture, Chinese meridian therapy, deep tissue massage, and herbal teas—have been used for hundreds, and in some cases thousands, of years. Why would they have lasted and been passed down from generation to generation unless they had some beneficial effect?

Why should you have to choose? I thought. How much more powerful to bring all the healing tools available into the examination room. So I evolved, slowly at first, then in a big jump when I accepted the position of medical director at the Paracelsus Clinic Lustmühle, which is located about an hour by train from the Zurich airport.

Nine of us at the clinic are licensed M.D.s. We also employ many nurses and three dentists and dental hygienists. Holistic dentistry is an important component of biological medicine. There is also a kinesiologist, an anthroposophical breathing therapist, masseuses, an acupuncturist, a psychologist, and an energy healer. Each of us followed a different path to arrive here; but for us all, disillusionment with the orthodox way and empirical experience with our patients over time led us to explore a wider universe of healing. While our medicine is often referred to as "alternative," we see it as the main road to good health.

My longtime association for over 25 years with biological medicine and for over 15 years with the Paracelsus Clinic has been happy. I've learned a great deal about healing, and I continue to learn—both from scientific studies and from my patients. My associates and I are not magicians. But it is immensely satisfying to see the tremendous number of people we help either to effect a complete cure or to manage difficult symptoms. The most fulfilling part is how we empower patients in the management of their own care. For Swiss biological medicine is a joint practice between doctor and patient. The sort of deep healing that Dr. Rau's Way offers can be truly successful only if the patient chooses to follow the path. With healing based on nutrition, a long-term commitment is required. On the other hand, knowing that you can—and indeed must—participate in improving your own health through the daily choices you make is extremely empowering.

Taking Control of Your Health

I remember spending a great deal of time with my father when I was a little boy. After World War II, times were hard in Europe; even Switzerland was poor, and public services and social support systems had not yet been established. Often, I'd listen to my father talking with his business colleagues or friends. Sooner or later, the conversation would invariably turn to their dreams for the future, their fervent desire that their children should have a better life than they had had. They wished for better schools, more economic opportunities, greater affluence, more ability to enjoy life, and so on.

At that point in the conversation, my father would always interrupt and ask pointedly, "And so, what are *you* doing to build a better world for your children?" He understood the power of personal responsibility and choice to make things happen. And what is powerful socially and professionally is equally powerful in terms of nutrition and health.

Whenever someone develops a serious illness or a chronic degenerative disease, his or her first question is, Why me? Guilt over illness is a misplaced emotion, and it can be destructive, because a positive outlook can influence the course of a disease by significantly boosting the immune response.

That is not to say that simply being happy and "good" will keep you disease free or cure you spontaneously. It simply means that to heal, it helps to marshal together all the positive forces of the self—body and soul.

Too often, I find that patients obsess over what they did or did not do earlier in their life. In the course of treating an illness, blame is not a helpful emotion. But a sense of personal responsibility is. Taking charge of your life and dealing forthrightly with your problems can greatly enhance your chances of effecting a cure. That's why nutrition, which is something you do have control over, is such an important part of Swiss biological medicine and is the basis of Dr. Rau's Way.

Only by understanding what led to the disease in your individual case can you work with your doctor in healing and in preventing a reoccurrence in the future. Simply swallowing a pill is never enough. That may relieve the outward manifestations of your problem, but it will not attack the root cause; sometimes it will actually make things worse. Symptoms may look alike from patient to patient, but the reasons they arise vary greatly. Even if you suppress symptoms like a headache or a fever, your illness will continue and worsen until you discover where it comes from and deal with the underlying cause or causes.

An Individualized Approach to Health

Everyone gets sick at one time or another. But different people develop different problems at different times, and they respond in different ways. One person might bounce back from the flu in a week, while another might be fatigued and listless for a month. One patient might respond swiftly to cancer treatments, while another might lose the battle despite all attempts to save him. That's because no matter how similar the outward symptom or manifestation of a disease, internally everyone is unique. One man may get a rash because he's allergic to strawberries, another because he has a subclinical infection from an old root canal. One woman gets a recurrent headache because her sinus passages are congenitally deformed; another because she has an allergy to wheat or to cow's milk.

Very often, we find hidden causes for chronic diseases in the teeth. Heavy metals from amalgam fillings and toxins from subclinical infections in old root canals are frequent causes of symptoms and impediments to healing. Even trace amounts of mercury in the system, for example, can lead to colitis, sinusitis, or asthma. Toxic root canals can lead to any number of problems, among them facial neuralgia, tinnitus, migraines, joint pain, and even cancer.

To effect a permanent solution, the symptom experienced by the patient needs an interpreter to divine its origin. Swiss biological medicine strives to diagnose and remove the underlying *cause*, or *causes*, of an ailment so that the symptoms are alleviated permanently and as naturally as possible, without drugs that damage the body. Our goal is to help you understand *why* you have a particular problem so that it can be vanquished with deep, natural healing.

Swiss biological medicine is holistic in that it sees each individual as unique and as a complete entity. As practiced at the Paracelsus Clinic, it strives to determine scientifically exactly why a particular individual is susceptible to a certain illness. That involves getting to know the individual well and understanding their history—lifestyle, environmental exposure, psychological profile—as well as their unique biochemistry and the way they lead their life. Complete physical examinations, detailed blood work, dental X-rays, and genetic testing where necessary yield many clues. Talking to patients and listening closely to what they have to say about themselves and their health is the doctor's most important tool. Only by thoroughly understanding the individual can you know how to treat them effectively.

Of course, the differences among people who are not seriously ill are less obvious. Further complicating the diagnostic process is the fact that a good deal of everyone's health is determined by the general internal condition of the body. But the beauty of Swiss biological medicine is that we pay so much attention to this inner environment, and that is the part over which *you* have control. Much of adjusting this internal milieu and regulating the body is done through nutrition, which is why this book can be so valuable to you. While you may or may not make it to a biological medicine clinic—though, of course, I hope you do someday for your own good—you can easily practice in your own home what I preach. And the benefits will accrue not only to you but to your entire family as well. The healthy eating described in my Maintenance Diet for Life (Chapter 8) is as excellent for children as it is for adults.

If you make a commitment to Dr. Rau's Way, it will change your body for sure: you will become more vital in many ways, both subtle and obvious. Over the longer term, it will also change *you*—your thinking, your interests, your mood, and your mental abilities. Alkaline individuals are "younger," more intuitive, more peaceful, as well as fitter, and more productive in their daily lives.

Many highly scientific studies have proven the effectiveness of emotional well-being and a strong, positive outlook in combating illness. A strong, vital physical structure strengthens the psyche as well. Think of the positive state of mind you have when you feel physically fit and energetic. Imagine the sense of emotional well-being you have when you are not plagued by pain and physical suffering. When we heal the body, we often find we heal the psyche as well.

Biological medicine also offers tremendous comfort to the patient by not only curing the complaint, but also determining the underlying cause of that complaint. The fear and anxiety that often accompany chronic illness are somewhat mitigated when patients don't have to agonize over why they feel the way they do. The effectiveness of my treatments lessens the likelihood that the pain and disabling symptoms will reoccur. There is nothing more depressing than spending your life anticipating the return of pain.

At the Paracelsus Clinic we employ a wide range of therapeutic treatments, but the most important treatment is one you can practice yourself at home: diet. That's why I developed Dr. Rau's Way.

CHAPTER TWO

The Healing Power of Food

Did you know that 80 percent of the adult immune defenses resides in the small intestine? In children, that percentage is even higher. With roughly 10,000 square feet of surface area, the intestinal tract maintains what is arguably the most intensive contact with the outside world of any other organ in the body. No wonder food affects us so much.

When you eat, some digestion, especially of starches, begins with saliva in the mouth. That's why it's so important to chew your food well—20 to 30 times—before swallowing. Then hydrochloric acid in your stomach liquefies the food so it can pass into the duodenum, where enzymes and gall fluid are added and protein digestion begins. At the same time, the body releases sodium bicarbonate in an effort to buffer the powerful acid. It's when the food passes into the small intestine, however, that the action really begins and nutrients are absorbed.

Bile, which is secreted by the liver, and pancreatic enzymes are both released into the small intestine upon demand at the proper stage of digestion. These chemicals, along with the good bacteria in your gut, attack the liquefied food from your stomach, breaking it down further into molecules small enough to pass through the thin intestinal walls so that they can be absorbed into the body. These molecules include glucose, which fuels all your cells; amino acids, which build proteins, important elements that contribute to cell integrity, healing, and growth; and lipids (or fats), which help carry fat-soluble vitamins into the body, regulate metabolism, act as storage for future energy, and feed the brain and neural system, among other functions.

There are literally trillions of bacteria cells in your intestines; that's ten times the number of "human" cells you have in your body. When those bacteria are the healthy kind, they act in conjunction with your intestinal system to process what you eat. Fiber from raw vegetables and whole grains, an alkaline balance achieved from a diet low in excess protein, and few environmental toxins keep these bacteria thriving and stimulate T cell (T lymphocyte) immunity and the lining of your gut.

WHY THE INTESTINAL BACTERIA ARE SO IMPORTANT

One reason Swiss biological medicine stresses nutrition so much is that your intestinal bacteria are responsible for the stimulation of much of your immune system . . . and more. They:

- Protect the intestinal mucous membranes essential for absorbing nutrients. *Think of this like the well-manicured lawn on a golf course.*

- Offer resistance against the growth of bad bacteria and fungi, like systemic yeast. *A properly cultivated lawn allows no weeds to grow.*

- Detoxify the body. *The bacteria act like blotting paper, soaking up environmental toxins, such as arsenic, before they can enter the body.*

- De-acidify the body. *Acid-building anaerobic bacteria do this by transporting organically bound acids from the body, depositing them in the stools for removal.*

- Produce highly unsaturated fatty acids, essential for maintenance of cell membranes, out of saturated or monounsaturated fatty acids.

It is in the passage through the filmy, very delicate walls of the small intestine and into the body that these molecules from your food first confront your immune system. Before reaching the liver, where they are metabolized and sent out to where they are needed, these molecules are vetted, as it were, by several structures, including one of the most important parts of your immune system: groups of tiny lymph glands, called Peyer's patches, which lie within the intestinal wall lining. Here, bad bacteria, foreign organisms, and any substances you are allergic to are filtered out.

It is also here in the gut where your acid/alkaline balance is established, partially by the intestinal bacteria, partially by the mucous membrane itself. For all these reasons, we must respect the truth of what Hippocrates, the first great doctor, said about health: "Let food be thy medicine."

Building a Better Body, Cell by Cell

We know from laboratory and epidemiological studies as well as from our own experience that at the core of much chronic degenerative disease is a problem with nutrition. At the Paracelsus Clinic, we use a comprehensive dietary program—Dr. Rau's Way—that we have found to be effective in restoring and maintaining the body's acid/alkaline balance, in strengthening immunity, and in curing disease.

But we prescribe my nutritional plan to all our patients, not just those with serious diseases. Because preventative medicine is the best medicine. And anyone looking to improve their general health, alleviate allergies, increase their energy, or even just plain look younger and better will benefit from healthy eating. It is as invigorating and rejuvenating as any tonic.

The fact is, what you do and do not eat has an effect on every cell in your body and on the fluids that flow around those cells. The goal is to choose foods that create an alkaline internal milieu, which allows good bacteria to propagate in the intestinal tract; give the body all the vitamins and minerals it needs to flourish; and nourish without an overload of protein, which clogs the system, acidifies the blood, and draws out calcium and other minerals from the bones and connective tissues. Then, as part of the natural cycle of regeneration, cells that are currently sick can be reborn as normal, healthy cells.

Since each cell in your body is constantly renewing itself, and organs are simply groups of dedicated cells, it seems reasonable that a sick organ, causing distressing symptoms, can, with proper encouragement, be made over—repopulated with new, healthy cells until it is essentially rebuilt. We strive to cure people or, perhaps more properly, help them achieve a balance of good health—even one cell at a time, if that is what it takes. That's why patience is sometimes required. Building a better body from the inside out usually takes time.

Dr. Rau's Way

Dr. Rau's Way gives you the tools to take control of your health. Good nutrition is as essential to health as oxygen. Changing the way you eat will affect you tremendously, whether you have a life-threatening disease, a chronic illness, a family propensity toward a particular problem, a wish to feel and look better than you do at present, or simply the desire to lose weight.

Dr. Rau's Way consists of a two-step dietary plan. The first stage is designed to transform your body, cell by cell, by detoxifying first—getting rid of excess and degraded proteins that clog the lymph and blood systems; by de-acidifying, which allows the body and metabolism to come into balance; by removing hidden food allergens, greatly boosting the immune system; and by nourishing the intestinal flora, which is key to all good health.

I call this three-week nutritional cleansing program, which can benefit almost everyone, *The Swiss Detox Diet*. This carefully calculated, vegetarian-based diet jump-starts your progress toward health, encourages

THE PHOENIX FACTOR:
HOW LONG IT TAKES FOR DIFFERENT CELLS
TO RENEW THEMSELVES

All organs regenerate themselves constantly. Our goal is to substitute healthy cells for weak or damaged cells. Providing the right nutrition helps create a healthier organ by establishing an optimal internal environment for at least one or more generation spans of the organ's cells—that is, to replace all the cells in an organ with new and better cells takes at least as much time as the life span of those cells. It is because it takes about 3 weeks for the intestinal bacteria to turn over that my Swiss Detox Diet takes 21 days.

Life Spans of Various Cells

BLOOD: ERYTHROCYTES (RED BLOOD CELLS) . . . . . . .1 month

LEUKOCYTES (WHITE BLOOD CELLS)

GRANULOCYTES . . . . .2 months

LYMPH CELLS . . . . .3 weeks

INTESTINAL BACTERIA . . . . .1 to 3 weeks

INTESTINAL MUCOUS MEMBRANES . . . . .2 to 4 weeks

LIVER . . . . .6 to 12 months

MUSCLES . . . . .4 to 18 months

SKIN . . . . .2 to 12 months

HEART ARTERIES . . . . .2 years

HEART MUSCLE . . . . .1 to 2 years

CARTILAGE . . . . .2 to 4 years

BONES . . . . .2 to 6 years

NERVES . . . . .2 to 7 years rapid weight loss where needed, and acts like a tonic in terms of energy and mental focus. Most importantly, it removes 90 percent of known food allergens.

The first week avoids not just dairy, but almost all gluten, as well. Raw and lightly steamed vegetables, a little fruit, nuts, seeds, and a few whole grains, along with vital oils comprise most meals. Hunger is not an issue. You may enjoy—in fact, are encouraged to have—two snacks a day, in addition to three regular meals. One of the delights of this plan is the way it keeps your blood sugar on a very even keel, which means your energy level stays high all day. This is an "up," exhilarating program, not a depressive diet of deprivation.

By the second week, you will already experience a difference in the way you feel. It may well astound you that nutrition can make such a big adjustment, not only to the body, but to the psyche. Often, people find that their spirits lift dramatically. This is a very good diet for people prone to depression. This second week, your eating opportunities open up dramatically. In addition to enjoying a wide variety of vegetables and fruits, more whole grains are added to the diet at this time as well as small amounts of rice and beans, an egg, and even a little goat and sheep cheese by the end of the week. Because more foods are allowed, the range of recipes opens up considerably, so that the pleasure of eating returns.

Week three remains vegetarian, but more sweetened treats are allowed along with more potatoes and sweet potatoes, legumes, a greater variety of whole grains, and sheep and goat dairy. You will not be bored if you follow the plan, and you will feel great.

This stage of the program consists of three short weeks, but if you have a diagnosed disease, chronic illness, or severe metabolic imbalance, you will benefit greatly by repeating the detox diet so that you follow it for a total of six weeks. For people who are seriously overweight or who have chronic high blood pressure, it is safe—and beneficial—for as long as three months.

If you're essentially healthy and simply want to stay that way, the three-week Swiss Detox Diet is probably all you need—21 days to get yourself into balance, before graduating to my Maintenance Diet for Life. The detox diet is especially good for cancer patients and others suffering from severe inflammatory and autoimmune diseases, and it's great for the cardiovascular system. The only people who should skip the initial detox are pregnant women and nursing mothers. Baby comes first! I encourage these women to go straight to "Maintenance."

The Maintenance Diet for Life is as much a beginning as it is an end. It presents a rich nutritional program that offers variety and complete sustenance along with everything you need to both sustain health and heal yourself for good. I don't want you to go through that wonderful detox program, lose 10 or 15 pounds, feel fresh and vital, and then return to the bad old ways. This diet, which keeps up the good work of the Swiss Detox Diet in a more moderate way, is designed to last a lifetime.

The eating plan itself is simple: essentially an extension and elaboration of the detox diet with many new foods added on, including a little fish and chicken. You must, however, approach the expanded diet with not only enthusiasm, but alertness. Because unless you visit a biological medicine clinic to be diagnosed for your individual food allergies, you will have to observe your responses closely each time a new food is tried to make sure you have no bad reactions. The goal is to continue to avoid hidden food allergies as well foods that contain toxins and additives. In the following chapters, I'll teach you how.

Later in the book, I'll also show you a way you can do a quick refresher course if you "fall off the wagon." I always tell my patients, "With Dr. Rau's Way, you cannot cheat." That's true in the sense that once your body is detoxified, deviating from my diet once in a while can't hurt you. But if you've been on a long trip or simply let yourself go over the holidays and you feel it, you can always jump into my One-Week Intensive Cure, a sort of modified fast, and then bounce right back into maintenance. This strict one-week diet is paired with our very effective Liver Cleanse, which significantly lightens your toxic load overnight and lays the groundwork for ongoing deep healing.

Before we get to details of the diet, let's follow up what you've just learned about biological medicine with a chapter that explains many of the treatments and therapies you will encounter if you decide to visit Paracelsus Clinic Lustmühle in Switzerland or any of the biological medicine clinics in the United States. Understanding some of these processes will also further explain why diet, especially acid/alkaline balance, is so important to a healthy internal environment.

CHAPTER THREE

A Catalog of Treatments

DIAGNOSTIC TOOLS AND THERAPIES
USED IN SWISS BIOLOGICAL MEDICINE

To better understand integrated Swiss biological medicine—as we practice it at the Paracelus Clinic in Lustmühle, Switzerland, and in our sister clinic at Al Ronc—it will help if you learn about some of our diagnostic procedures and treatments. A number of these can be found in biological clinics across the United States. And some important aspects of our method of healing can be—and must be—practiced in your own home. Perhaps you have already experienced some of these therapies or you are embarking upon a course of biological medicine cures. Even if your goal is simply to improve your health by diet through following Dr. Rau's Way, the information in this chapter will help you understand who we are and what we do.

Doctor–Patient Interview

Anyone who suffers from a chronic illness knows just how difficult it is to get help. If all you had to do was pick up the phone, make an appointment, and get taken care of, being sick wouldn't be so much work. But in this world of deductibles, co-pays, and referrals, not to speak of lobbying and consumer advertising by pharmaceutical companies, health care is not as simple as it once was. The average amount of time a doctor in group practice spends with a patient is seven minutes. Really, how much do you think can be accomplished in seven minutes?

The average examination at the Paracelsus Clinic lasts about 30 minutes. I devote a significant portion of my examination just listening, talking to, and observing a patient before I even begin my physical examination. I ask a number of questions that sometimes puzzle my patients but that give me invaluable hidden information. I'm more interested in their experience of their symptoms rather than the findings determined by other doctors and tests, because Swiss biological medicine looks at disease in a completely different way.

In this important initial consultation, I often learn as much about a person as from any number of subsequent tests. If I am open to my patients, their aura of energy or lack thereof, their complexion, body language, intellectual vigor, attitude toward their health, and list of complaints give me key information on an intuitive as well as a technical level. I gather the best set of clues imaginable so that I can begin my scientific investigation in the right direction.

A manual palpation is also an important part of my exam because it tells me a great deal about a person's vitality and physical condition. I'm surprised at the stories I hear from patients about the arm's-length treatment they frequently receive at other doctors' offices.

Often, a patient will say, "Dr. Rau just knows what's wrong with me." But, in fact, it is nothing more than paying attention and feeling, and sometimes also seeing, the warmth and energy that radiates from a body and of understanding what those signals mean.

Unfortunately, in formal medical education this combination of natural intuition and human sensibilities is often lost. Too often, doctors let themselves be steered by cold technical findings, which are generalizations, rather than looking closely at the individual right before them. To avoid this bias, I always examine a patient without any preconceptions or prejudices. Only after this first evaluation do I read the laboratory reports and technical findings they have brought along.

But this initial interview works both ways. Not only do I take in a great deal about the person across the desk from me, but I also give of myself to the patient. My energy, empathy, and certainty of the good results that will ensue when we work together are very consciously offered up to the person who has come to me. This is not unique to me but is part of the humanistic approach integral to Swiss biological medicine. Only a doctor who is full of dedication to his or her work, who lives in a harmony with the earth, and who loves his patients can truly empathize with those who need help. What we have to offer is not only our scientific "bag of tricks," but perhaps the most important ingredient of all: hope.

A positive state of mind is not hocus-pocus; it gives a major boost to the immune system, which is a good way to begin the healing process. Many studies have proven the importance of hope, love, and support to survival, especially when an illness is critical or chronic. The biological medical doctor offers his hand in trust to the patient who is ready to make the journey to health. Then the technical investigation begins.

The variety of diagnostic procedures and biological medicine treatments offered under one roof at Paracelsus Clinic Lustmühle distinguishes it from many other healing facilities. Since our theories teach us that many serious and chronic debilitating diseases often have more than one origin, this diversity is extremely important. The array of therapies at our disposal offers us the most effective way to treat an illness from several different directions at the same time.

Diagnostic Tools Used in
Swiss Biological Medicine

Darkfield Microscopy

This is a fancy name for looking at a slide of blood viewed under a microscope with a very high power magnification (1200×), which is backlit in a special way so light flows through the sample. This allows us to see not only the individual blood cells, but much smaller bodies, which are not visible in normal hematology slides.

Darkfield microscopy is an immensely valuable tool that allows us to graphically view the state of the patient's internal environment. It reveals overacidity of the blood, infections, internal stresses, and tendencies to develop circulatory illnesses, problems relating to imbalances of the intestinal tract, and malign degenerative diseases, including cancer.

It's usually the first test we do, and it is one of my favorite diagnostic techniques because it gives me so much information about a patient in a graphic and dynamic format. I can read a great deal about the state of a person's health in a single drop of her blood. A painless prick of the earlobe—in the United States it's more common to use the fingertip—yields a drop or two of live—i.e., fresh—blood. The sample is sandwiched between two glass plates, and the slide is viewed several times, which helps us judge the stress tolerance of the cells.

The first examination occurs immediately, while the blood is still fluid. This reveals a great deal about the state of the patient's internal environment: acid/alkaline balance, current infections, propensity toward malignancy, and level of vitality. Then the blood is viewed at least one more time after it has dried completely and sometimes at intervening stages. The dried blood also yields a portrait—this time of possible toxic overload with heavy metals and other environmental stresses as well as indications of bad bacteria and parasites.

Like a meteorologist viewing a weather chart, the information I see not only tells me a great deal about the patient's physical condition at the moment, but allows me to predict what may likely happen to him medically in the future. A major advantage of this sensitive tool is the diagnostic edge it gives us over traditional methods. This "early warning" alerts us to the development of some diseases—such as rheumatoid arthritis, colitis, and chronic eczema—at a stage in which much damage can be averted and treatment can be much more effective.

Thermography

We use two types of thermography: contact and infrared.

Like Darkfield blood analysis, **computer regulation thermography (CRT)** is another highly sensitive technique we use for measuring deep internal problems at an early stage. Readings are taken with a special contact thermometer that measures skin temperature at 119 different points on the body, each of which corresponds to a specific organ, gland, or tissue. The patient is left disrobed in a cool room for 10 minutes. This stimulates the body to try and regulate itself. Then a second reading of the same points is taken. These results are fed into a computer system and compared against millions of findings to yield diagnostic information. If the reactive capacity (the ability to recover) is diminished in any way, the temperature at the skin point will reflect it. These results reflect old or acute blockages, disturbances, inflammations, and even cancer at an early stage.

Infrared thermography is now being used, especially in Europe, to detect early cancer. It is noninvasive and exposes the patient to none of the radiation of traditional X-ray screening. A large, joint American-German study done with breast cancer patients determined that, compared to standard X-ray mammography, infrared thermography—also called thermal imaging or infrared imaging—was highly accurate in detecting early-stage breast cancer.

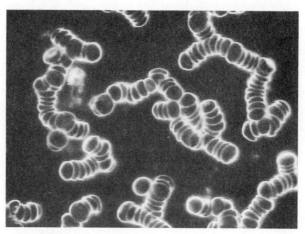

The first photograph shows typical *rouleaux*, snakelike clumps of red blood cells (erythrocytes), which indicate an acidic internal environment, usually caused by hyperproteinization.

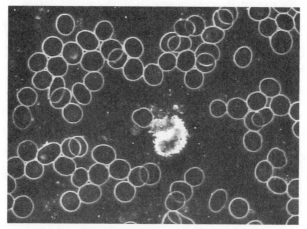

The second photograph illustrates red blood cells in a healthy, alkaline environment: cells are free-flowing and cell walls are thinner.

Traditional Blood Work

We also do a complete blood analysis, similar to the kind you would receive from a traditional allopathic doctor, but much more thorough. Not only do we check cholesterol, liver enzymes, and thyroid function, we test for all kinds of heavy metals, trace elements, old viruses, and environmental toxins as well as imbalances that may be affecting a patient's health or that may be a sign of a disease. A lack of certain hormones—the substances that regulate not only sexual, but all metabolic functions—or of highly unsaturated fatty acids is a frequent cause of neurological problems and diseases of the immune system.

Hair Mineral Analysis (HMA)

Chemical analysis of hair is particularly helpful in showing the presence of heavy metals, such as lead and aluminum. When we find this kind of contamination, we institute several forms of chelation therapy to rid the body of these poisons. (Note: Mercury binds more strongly with internal tissues, so HMA is not the most reliable tool for detecting it. We test for mercury in other ways and use several therapies for purging it from the body: chelation and special heavy-metal draining infusions.)

HMA is primarily helpful because it shows specific patterns, such as damage to the intestines from food allergies (so-called "leaky gut syndrome") and bone loss. It can also detect attention deficient and distress syndrome (ADDS), which is a neurological toxicity that is, by the way, nearly always connected to high aluminum contamination. Aluminum is mainly ingested because it binds with fluorides in water, salt, and dental treatments.

Heart-Rate Variability

The very delicate measurements recorded by the simple heart-rate variability test give us a great deal of information about the subtle balance between the parasympathetic and sympathetic nervous systems, which together coordinate all automatic, or unconscious, physical reactions, like breathing, heart rate, and digestion. This is the only test that measures the strength of the unconscious nervous system. Furthermore, the results show graphically how the body reacts to an irritation, helping us to decide on the best course of treatment.

A patient's pulse is taken both lying down and standing up over a period of several minutes. Variations provide many clues about the reactive capability and healing power of a patient. We often use this in cases of chronic stress and fatigue, but it also indicates the propensity toward degenerative diseases and even cancer. A second testing after treatments are given offers a good way to measure the effectiveness of those treatments.

Therapies Used in
Swiss Biological Medicine

Infusions

These are given intravenously in a special patented saline solution. Our saline solution is completely different from that made from sodium chloride, which is used in most Western medical facilities. Ours is composed of sodium bicarbonate and sodium chlorine, blended in a very special way that makes it isotonic, or easily absorbed by cells. Consequently, it deacidifies the body through the bloodstream in an extremely efficient fashion. In addition to the saline, we add different remedies to the infusion, which vary greatly depending upon the patient's individual problems, but often include high doses of vitamin C and the B vitamins, including folic acid, in addition to isopathic remedies.

Ozone Therapy

We also use these infusion sessions to practice ozone therapy. This involves removing 100 ml (roughly ½ cup) of blood, saturating it with ozone, and then returning it to the patient through the intravenous line. This increases the oxygen uptake of all cells, refreshing the tissues, speeding up cell metabolism, and, consequently, facilitating healing.

Acupuncture, Chinese Meridian Theory, and the Five-Element Model

The Chinese practice of acupuncture goes back more than 4,000 years. A textbook that codified much ancient information was first published in China in the early seventeenth century, and it is still used in Chinese medical schools today. Even Western doctors have acknowledged the immense usefulness of acupuncture for relieving pain and alleviating inflammation, especially from arthritis. In fact, many traditional insurance plans will pay for acupuncture.

Acupuncture's effectiveness is based on opening up energy pathways that have been charted throughout the body. These pathways correspond to pairs of organs that are grouped according to different characteristics the Chinese ascribe to five elements: earth, metal, water, wood, and fire. These, in turn, relate to different psychological or emotional models of character. While it sounds alchemical, like other medical systems, it is a model—one that can be very useful for descriptive and diagnostic purposes.

Neural Therapy

My technique of neural therapy takes acupuncture a step further. It stimulates the unconscious (parasympathetic) nervous system by injecting very specific acupuncture points with correlating homeopathic and isopathic remedies. By using the Chinese meridians to pinpoint spots on the body, particularly around vital organs, we can inject these remedies where they will do the most good, delivering them not just to the bloodstream, but to key spots where they are needed. We often get dramatic results with these injections, which can last for weeks or even months; sometimes they provide a permanent cure by improving the body's healing capacity.

Panoramic Dental X-ray and Holistic Dental Treatments

Holistic dentistry has long been an important part of integrated Swiss biological medicine. Infections, sometimes buried in the gums, and toxicity from heavy metal contamination from amalgam fillings are of particular concern. Sometimes these foci, as we call these toxic disturbances, give us clues to healing patients whose conditions have had us stumped. In fact, the relationship between problematic teeth and diseased organs is so strong that our dentist can frequently tell just from the X-ray what physical problem the patient has. By removing dead teeth and cleaning out all the tissues around them, we often effect cures that have been eluding us for some time.

Hyperthermia Treatments

High-heat treatments—whole body as well as localized (Indiba)—are used to treat tumors, autoimmune diseases, and degenerative diseases such as osteoarthritis. Cancer cells cannot tolerate heat nearly as well as normal cells, so tumor patients in particular benefit from these hyperthermia sessions. Such intense heat also boosts the body's own defense mechanisms, encouraging proliferation of immune lymph cells and macrophages—large white blood cells you could think of as combination garbage collectors and policemen: they consume wasted and degraded proteins and kill cancer cells. Macrophages also target and ingest bad bacteria. For arthritis patients, the fever-induced state provides more metabolic power to the body, strengthening the up-building forces.

The temperature of patients undergoing these intense sessions with infrared light can rise as high as 104 degrees F. For safety, each patient is constantly monitored by both a doctor and a nurse, who are present in the room throughout the entire procedure. Some people endure the treatment because they know it will help them; others find it pleasurable and activating.

Liver Cleanse

Most people think toxins are eliminated from their body in sweat and urine, but actually most are discharged in bile from the liver that empties into the stools. The Liver Cleanse takes advantage of this by prescribing a special vegetarian diet with a great deal of apple juice, which opens up the bile ducts and allows the liver to drain freely, emptying itself of excess cholesterol and waste proteins. At Paracelsus Lustmühle and at our sister clinic, Al Ronc, we offer a weeklong detoxifying program built around the power of the Liver Cleanse. The diet is aided with colonic cleansing, local hyperthermia, and neural therapy to the liver as well as relaxation therapies. It's a great way to rejuvenate your body, detoxify, and prepare for healing. Chapter 11 details how to perform the Liver Cleanse at home.

Colonic Cleansing

A thorough but mild cleansing of the large intestine, accompanied by a gentle abdominal massage that stimulates the parasympathetic nervous system, cleans out toxins and bad bacteria, strengthens the immune system, and encourages the development of beneficial bacteria. At our clinics, we always accompany colonics with a specific reflorestation of intestinal flora. (Note: Of course, there are enemas you can take at home, but deep colonic cleansing should be done only by a licensed medical professional under controlled conditions. Well-meaning amateurs can do serious harm.)

Infrared Sauna

This unique tool allows us to use high heat in a more concentrated way. It focuses energy to within millimeters to reach the lymph system and stimulate it with heat, which boosts the healing power of the immune system. It also increases the circulation within the fat just under the skin so that fat-soluble toxins are freely released.

Myoreflex Therapy

Myoreflexology is a type of osteopathy—that is, the branch of medicine that attributes certain illnesses to misalignment of muscles, ligaments, tendons, and bones. (In the United States, doctors of osteopathy [D.O.s] often hold practices that are similar to those of M.D.s.) It integrates acupuncture points and meridian theory. Treatment involves a kind of pressure-point massage that moves energy along the fascia meridians—energy pathways that run throughout the body—and dramatically opens up the function of nerves, muscles, and connective tissue. Long-term treatment has shown positive results with paralysis. Paracelsus Swiss biological medicine also uses many different kinds of massage to relax the patient and alleviate pain.

Vitamin and Mineral Supplements

Proper nutrients are essential to healthy intestinal flora and to metabolization of all the amino acids. Absence of proper vitamins and minerals leads to imbalances that cause a variety of ills. Because some diseases and genetic flaws use up excessive amounts of these nutrients or block their uptake, a potent supplement is good insurance.

Isopathic, Homeopathic, and Chinese Herbal Remedies

Here are three completely different sorts of remedies we employ for a range of purposes. Isopathic remedies, manufactured by the Sanum company and available through biological and naturopathic doctors, are designed to downgrade pathogenic microorganisms in the blood, disarming bacteria and viruses by pairing up with them and neutralizing them—a little like antimatter annihilating matter.

Homeopathic preparations work the opposite way; they are predicated on like curing like, in very dilute solutions. For example, if you have a rash

from poison ivy, the homeopathic solution would contain the active inflammatory element in poison ivy diluted to a completely benign, almost
undetectable level. The homeopathic solution stimulates the same response
in the immune system as the active poison ivy, helping to effect a cure.

At Paracelsus, we have developed specific kinds of homeopathic
preparations, called *nosodes,* which are exceptionally effective. These contain the information from old diseases and viral infections from the patient in a homeopathic dilution. They often produce truly amazing
results, especially with arthritis and neurological problems.

Chinese herbal teas and potions have proven extremely effective in
treating many systemic problems. At wellness centers across the United
States, nurses caring for chemotherapy patients frequently recommend
them to Chinese herbal healers, whose tisanes combat the nausea and fatigue that accompany such treatment. We use Chinese herbs for many
purposes.

Note: All these cures work naturally in harmony with the body. Except
in rare cases of critical emergency, biological medicine does not espouse
the use of pharmaceutical drugs, which harm the body's natural immune
system and disarm the individual's natural ability to fight off disease. Often
Swiss biological medicine treatments practiced over time remove the need
for traditional medicines or allow the dosage to be reduced.

Surgery and Chemotherapy and/or Radiation: Where Necessary to Stop the Clock

At the Paracelsus Clinic in Lustmühle, we offer an advanced tumor treatment program, which has enjoyed notable success, particularly with early-
stage breast and prostate cancers. Our biological treatments are conducted
along with orthodox treatments or in between courses of chemotherapy
to bolster the body and help repair some of the damage done by the poisons, which destroy many healthy cells along with the tumors. Surgery,
chemotherapy, and radiation are used when absolutely necessary to stop
the tumor so we can buy the time we need to let the patient heal from

within—but always in conjunction with intensive biological medicine treatments. In my experience, it is because we not only treat the cancer, but also its underlying causes, that I see the incidence of recurrence as lower than with conventional treatment.

Psychological Counseling

Chronic disease almost invariably engenders strong emotional responses, sometimes even depression and despair. Fear goes hand in hand with a bad prognosis. Since a positive outlook not only makes the patient feel better, but also significantly boosts the immune system, talking about illness and regaining hope is of paramount importance. Wherever appropriate, we encourage family participation.

There is one treatment we have not yet discussed, even though it forms the basis of all healing: diet. We offer it at the clinic; yet it is one of the few—though most powerful—techniques you can practice yourself at home by following Dr. Rau's Way. In the next chapter, you'll learn what my nutritional program consists of and why it is such powerful medicine.

CHAPTER FOUR

Dr. Rau's Way

HEALING THROUGH DIET AND NUTRITION

My medicine is simple: Like a good organic farmer tending soil in a garden, my goal is to nourish the basic substances of the body in every way possible, but primarily through diet, so that all the nutrients you need for good health are absorbed and used as efficiently as possible. This causes your natural defenses to grow strong and flourish. In the end, it is your own body that does the work. Think of this process as "deep healing."

Just as the condition of the fields determines the quality of the farmer's crops, so the internal environment of the human body determines a person's health. If the soil is poor, even the finest heirloom vegetable cannot grow well. But if the soil is rich and well watered, even a weak plant can thrive. If your internal environment is corrupted, despite a strong genetic constitution, you may fall ill. But if your body is nourished, cared for properly, and fed the right vitamins, minerals, trace elements, and correct balance of foods, even someone with a vulnerable constitution can heal and be well.

When I was a schoolboy, we did an interesting experiment in school. We dug up a square foot of rich grassy soil, including the roots, from the schoolyard and transplanted it to the forest. Then we dug up a section of the forest floor and similarly transplanted it to the schoolyard. One year later, you could not tell where we had planted our squares of soil—neither in the forest nor in the schoolyard. The local environment had taken over.

So it is with your body. It's how you care for your own internal environment—especially your intestinal flora, lymph system, and blood—by the nutrition you feed it over the long term that makes such a big difference in how your organs and immune system function and, consequently, in your overall health.

That's why deep healing makes so much sense. How could human beings have evolved through the ages if they did not possess this biological resilience? Think how the world has changed over the past few hundred, not to speak of thousands, of years. Imagine the new chemicals we've been exposed to, diseases that have arisen, environmental pollution that has come and gone. Without the ability to adapt and heal, there would be no human race.

Each of us has a powerful defense department built right into our bodies. We all possess biological mechanisms that search out and destroy invading enemies; these cells are designed to target and obliterate mutant aberrations that threaten the established order. We also have fortifications and reserves that compensate for short-term weaknesses, whether from nutrition or from stress. Only a tremendous overload of harmful factors can disarm these formidable internal weapons. Yet as we age, we build up a substantial backlog of deleterious experiences. You could say, "Living is hazardous to your health." When we are born, most of us are healthy and pure in the sense of being untouched by the outside world. Subsequent exposure to all kinds of infections, poisons, harmful drugs, environmental pollution, and poor nutrition—even the act of aging—accumulates physically and psychically like sediment, clogging our body's ability to heal itself. These blockages and impediments to healing are what we call your "toxic load."

Rather than offering only temporal relief from a superficial symptom, Swiss biological medicine, practiced over time, offers a permanent cure for any number of chronic inflammatory and degenerative diseases by reducing this toxic load as much as possible. Long-term good nutrition acts like a vaccine to ward off many illnesses, including colds and flu. And for conditions for which no standard medicine is powerful enough to completely cure, Dr. Rau's Way coupled with other biological medicine treatments can greatly ameliorate symptoms; relieve suffering; and, in dire cases, delay—sometimes for many years—what is ultimately inevitable.

The secret of the power of my natural medicine is that it works on such a deep internal level that everyone benefits. This includes:

- People who are essentially well but perhaps are reaching those years when energy begins to wane and for whom avoiding illness takes on real meaning. They want to feel and look better than they have in years.

- People who are suffering either from chronic problems like migraine headaches, acid reflux, and allergies, which traditional treatments have not improved or have only suppressed, or who have vague but debilitating symptoms their doctors do not know how to recognize or treat.

- People who are fighting serious, even life-threatening, chronic inflammatory and degenerative diseases, such as cancer, rheumatoid arthritis, and MS.

Dr. Rau's Way works so well for such a broad range of disturbances because it nurtures the body at a very basic level through all the vital internal fluids, the intestinal bacteria, and the immune system to build a better body cell by cell, day by day.

That's why I see the healthy eating that promotes good health as an ongoing way of life—essential at certain critical moments when illness strikes but equally important to maintain even when you feel perfectly well. Because the right nutrition not only helps promote healing, it is in large part the best preventative medicine there is.

To allow good nutrition to do its work, however, we must blast away the toxic load, which acts as a blockage, preventing the deep healing from taking place. That's why my dietary plan is divided into two stages. First you have to detoxify your body and clean out all the decay and debris down to the bedrock. Next you must replace the soil, nourishing it with the right organic matter—the proper foods—and add fertilizer—vitamins, minerals, and natural remedies. Only then can real healing begin.

Dr. Rau's Way of healing through nutrition is simple. It:

DETOXIFIES first to expel as many toxins as possible in a short amount of time. By restricting protein intake strictly for 7 days and moderately for the next 14, by avoiding foods that tend to provoke hidden allergic reactions (especially cow dairy products), and by making sure you pump plenty of liquids through your system, the Swiss Detox Diet goes a long way toward lightening the toxic overload that led to your problem(s) in the first place. The high-fiber, low-calorie diet rids the body of excess fat, old degraded proteins, and other toxins, preparing your body for up-building and healing.

REGULATES your body in two ways: The diet restores an alkaline balance and relieves the stress of food allergies. All the good leafy greens and healthy oils called for support the intestinal flora. While you're absorbing the many vitamins and minerals you need to maintain good health, it is the fiber from fruits, vegetables, and whole grains combined with some healthful oils, such as olive oil, which nourish the good bacteria in your gut, boost your immune system, and strengthen all your internal healing powers.

MAINTAINS the important work of de-acidifying and avoiding food allergens while feeding and strengthening the immune system. Because cells are continually regenerating and some systems have a turnover life span of months, if not years, the plan is most effective over time. Repairing clogged arteries, for example, takes a minimum of two years.

At this maintenance stage, your dietary choices expand tremendously. You can enjoy a wide variety of foods, including chicken and fish along with fruits and vegetables, which continue to provide you with the widest range of vitamins, minerals, and other nutrients. My easy-to-follow maintenance diet is designed to be satisfying as well as nourishing. It helps you identify your own food allergies and provides a way of eating you can follow for the rest of your life.

What may be a bit misleading is the term *maintenance*. It sounds passive, whereas in truth, it is extremely active. Because this excellent nutrition *practiced over time* has a tremendous regenerative effect, it is up to you to continually choose the path toward improving your own health.

The Phoenix Factor

When you nurture your internal body, you optimize the rebuilding power that lies within every human being. As I have already explained, all living tissues renew within a certain period of time. If you have an organ that is sick, slowly degenerating, or not functioning as it should and you want to improve your health, you need to create a new organ that functions better. You do this by nourishing the internal environment that surrounds and sustains that organ, so that over time, cell by cell, you grow a better body, essentially optimizing your natural potential for healing.

That is, *if* we make the right choices and assume active personal responsibility for our own health, we can improve our quality of life. If you want a healthier body with more vigorous new cells replacing the old degenerating and diseased ones, *you* have to make the changes: in nutrition, attitude, and activity. And you have to continue to make these good choices over the long term to allow the tissues of your body to renew themselves.

While the biochemical reasons my diet heals are immensely complex, on the surface they can be viewed through a simple template. Dr. Rau's Way is designed to:

- Detoxify
- De-acidify
- Remove food allergens

- Enhance cellular metabolism
- Boost your immune system
- Regenerate weak or diseased organs

A Review of the Program

To amplify on these ideas, let's run through the complete program again. Dr. Rau's Way presents a dietary plan that encompasses two stages:

Stage 1: The Swiss Detox Diet

The Swiss Detox Diet, which lasts for a minimum of three weeks, is the centerpiece of Dr. Rau's Way. This powerful diet cleanses the body, purging old toxins while promoting deep healing through several channels. Biological medicine is based on a natural regulation of the body in terms of good bacteria in the intestines and the correct acid/alkaline balance of the blood, lymph system, and interstitial fluids. An overacidic internal environment causes many illnesses and metabolic flaws.

Two important ways to detox are to remove excess protein from the diet and to eliminate all food allergies—no simple task, especially because most people are not even aware of what their allergies are. Yet the Swiss Detox Diet, which is strictly vegetarian among other things, accomplishes both. In addition, it continues to lighten the toxic load that has built up over a lifetime.

This specially tailored nutritional plan must be followed over a course of at least three weeks and is most effective when adhered to for six weeks. It alleviates many physical stress factors. For one thing, it is a strong anti-allergy program because it eliminates 90 percent of the most common food allergens, which in itself clears up many troublesome symptoms. These hidden allergies are most damaging over time, as they have a cumulative effect, and they are silently responsible for a great deal of inflammation and congestion.

At the same time, the Swiss Detox Diet supports and nurtures three major biological systems that share a great deal of information among themselves and that are vital to good health: the gastrointestinal system, the circulatory system, and the immune system. Restricting protein consumption and correcting hyperacidity in the body helps rebuild healthy flora throughout the digestive tract, speeds up cellular metabolism, and gives a big boost to the body's natural immune system.

Meals on the Swiss Detox Diet are light yet satisfying; there's no sense of deprivation. Some of the foods permitted at this stage can, during the second and third weeks, be eaten in unlimited amounts, and hunger is not an issue. Because what good is a diet if you can't stay on it?

In a nutshell, beginning at week two, you can eat all the raw, steamed, and lightly sautéed vegetables you want, especially leafy greens, such as spinach, kale, and Swiss chard. These last are high in valuable omega-3 essential fatty acids, and they provide a rich source of vitamins, trace elements, and minerals, especially iron and calcium. That's why you need so little meat and dairy as a source for these nutrients. The truth is that vegetarians have measurably stronger bones and higher oxygenation of their red blood cells than meat-eaters.

You can—and should—eat many other vegetables, such as potatoes, carrots, beets, avocados, green beans, and corn as well as sprouts, seeds, chestnuts, and small amounts of legumes—many of which are rich in essential amino acids. You should have plenty of whole grains, with the exception of wheat, which is an allergen in many people. This means avoiding even whole wheat bread, pasta, and wheat flour–based sauces; during this time, spelt is a good substitute. While it is an older variety of wheat, it causes far fewer allergies.

Only from variety can you ensure you get all the amino acids, vitamins, minerals, and trace elements you need. Variety means enjoying at least two or three different vegetables or vegetables and a grain at each meal. It's best not to mix grains because this causes digestive problems in many people.

Roughage—that is, indigestible fiber—from these vegetables and from seeds and whole grains maintains the health and vitality of your intestinal flora. The ideal goal to reach is 50 percent of your dietary intake from raw vegetables, because the insoluble fiber helps eliminate old fats and proteins and nourishes your good intestinal bacteria. It also fills you up before you take in too many calories—a great boon when you're trying to lose weight. But 50 percent is a bit high for most people at first and might lead to gas or mild diarrhea. It should be considered an ideal to attain only gradually. You may want to strive for 25 or 30 percent in the beginning. Like the practice of yoga, healing is not a contest. Whatever is the right level for you at the moment is where you should be. Then you can reach a little farther each week.

The Swiss Detox Diet, which acts like a tonic, has a dramatic effect on metabolism and energy levels. It is, indeed, rejuvenating. It is not arbitrary that the minimum length of this stage of the program is 21 days: Three weeks are key because that is a natural cycle for the cellular turnover of the intestinal lymph cells (T lymphocytes), which are arguably the most important part of the immune system.

Most people feel the increased energy within three to five days. After ten days, the renewed vitality kicks in so powerfully it may amaze you. If you have a serious illness or feel you need more time at this stage, you are encouraged to repeat the three-week diet. Following it for six, or even nine weeks, in most cases, is not only well tolerated, but results in tremendous health benefits I will detail a little later.

Stage 2: Maintenance Diet for Life

The Maintenance Diet for Life is an easy-to-follow nutritional plan that is not a formal diet in the traditional sense; there is no counting involved, and while portion control of protein remains essential, many other foods can be enjoyed in any amounts you like. The program offers a healthy way to eat on an ongoing basis in order to prevent illness and maintain optimum health and vigor. You shouldn't be on a diet one month and off it the next. This is the way you should eat for the rest of your life.

IS DR. RAU'S WAY A WEIGHT-LOSS PROGRAM?

It is important to keep in mind that this is a way of eating designed primarily to improve health. It was not created as a weight-loss diet.

Nonetheless, because these menus regulate metabolism, people who are overweight will find they shed pounds effortlessly, and anyone underweight because of illness or poor nutrition will put on pounds and discover renewed vitality. When coupled with moderate exercise, such as walking 20 to 30 minutes a day, your metabolism will resolve itself to its optimum set point—where your body is in a healthy balance.

What's particularly good about using the Swiss Detox Diet for weight loss, aside from all the other health benefits that will ensue, is that while some diets are so severe that they caution you against staying on them for too long, this extremely effective diet can be maintained easily for up to three months. All it will do is continue to improve your health. Then when you switch to my Maintenance Diet for Life, you will not regain the pounds you lost, as often happens with other diets. In fact, if properly tailored to your needs, you can continue to lose weight even while enjoying a much broader assortment of foods.

At this stage, you'll continue to enjoy lots of organic fresh fruits and vegetables as well as whole grains and some sheep and goat dairy products. You'll be adding in a greater variety of grains, including a modicum of wheat. If you tolerate it well, imported semolina pasta is allowed. You may have chicken or fish two or three times a week as well as an egg once or twice. Because you've just gone through a detox program to cleanse your body and give your immune system a rest by removing a wide range of food allergies, you want to preserve all the good you've accomplished. Adding new ingredients to your diet slowly, one by one, and paying close attention to the effect of each food you eat will teach you what foods do and do not suit you. Remember, each individual is different. Chapter 11 explains all about food allergies—how to spot them and how to avoid them permanently.

THERE'S NO CHEATING!

One extra bonus of Dr. Rau's Way is that it is *impossible to cheat*. That's because once you have been on my Maintenance Diet for Life for a few months, it doesn't matter if you eat something forbidden when you go out to dinner or when you have guests over, or whenever you feel like a splurge. Assuming your health is not in a critical state—in which case you owe it to yourself to be strict—if you maintain the diet most of the time, falling off the wagon for one night will make no difference to your health at all. So there's no guilt and no stress.

And if you go on vacation or a business trip and find you've totally lost it for many days—or even for a couple of weeks—when you come home, you can jump back quickly by doing my One-Week Intensive Cure, which, especially if coupled with our excellent Liver Cleanse, will put you right back in balance.

Once you've established your baseline level of comfort with different foods and you get your kitchen set up (see Chapter 9), this way of eating involves less preparation time than much traditional cooking and allows plenty of appealing choices each day. Remember, a key aspect of the program is not only what you *cannot* eat but also all the things you *must* eat for good health.

While some foods, such as wholesome fresh fruits and vegetables, are mandatory and others, such as cow dairy products, are prohibited, there is a wide range of enticing foods to choose from—all good for your health. The plan is both simple to follow and highly appetizing. You'll never go hungry. In addition to three meals a day, one or two light snacks between meals are encouraged to make sure your blood sugar levels remain stable.

The good nutrition described by my eating plan regulates weight, maintains blood sugar levels throughout the day, and promotes overall vitality, physical vigor, and clarity of mind. It also acts as a buffer to slow the inevitable degeneration of aging, helping you look and feel as good as you can for as long as possible.

In point of practice, Dr. Rau's Way is a nutritional plan that is much more inclusive than restrictive. And once you're past the first week of the Swiss Detox Diet, amounts of many foods are virtually unlimited, so there is no feeling of self-denial or lack of pleasure at the dining table. That's why the menus and recipes at the end of this book were designed to be not just "correct," but also delicious. It's essential the diet be sustainable over time.

Of course, if you are critically ill, worried about a debilitating degenerative disease, or in between courses of chemotherapy, what you dine on may not be of the greatest importance. Comfort and ease of digestion are primary in these cases. In this context, it's easy to view food as medicine. Many of the recipes you'll find later in the book have been taken from the food served in the fine dining room of the Hotel Säntis in Teufen, the hotel that supports our clinic and where most of our patients stay. So you can be sure you will find them both delicious and easy to digest.

FOODS YOU *MUST* EAT ON THE MAINTENANCE DIET

- **Plenty of raw and lightly cooked leafy greens; root vegetables; other vegetables,** such as green beans and peas; and **fruits**—fresh, organic, and in season whenever possible. Include lots of these nutritious foods every day. These provide the bulk of the diet, because they contain fiber and lots of vitamins and minerals, and some proteins. With few exceptions, they metabolize alkaline, so they also de-acidify the body as well as increasing hormones and cellular metabolism.

- **Whole grains,** such as spelt, oats, quinoa, and amaranth, for protein, fiber, vitamins, and minerals.

- **At least 2 tablespoons of good fats,** such as olive oil, sunflower oil, flax seed oil, sesame oil, pumpkin seed oil, and grape seed oil, every day. (Note: Only olive oil and sunflower oil should be used for cooking.)

- **2 to 3 liters of uncarbonated, nonchlorinated spring water and herbal teas** daily between meals.

FOODS YOU *MAY* HAVE ON THE MAINTENANCE DIET

- **Basmati rice,** jasmine rice, and Arborio rice; brown rice, if you tolerate it

- **Imported semolina pasta** once or twice a week, if you tolerate gluten

- **Goat's and sheep's milk yogurt and cheeses,** such as Roquefort, Manchego, or Pecorino Romano, in small amounts several times a week

- **Freshly squeezed fruit juices:** only a 4-ounce glass in the morning, preferably with the pulp included

- **Egg:** one 3-minute egg twice a week

- **Organic soy products** once or twice a week

- **Beans and other legumes,** especially chickpeas and lentils, several times a week as a garnish, once or twice a week as a side dish

- **Organic, free-range chicken or turkey, or healthful fish:** small portions two or three times a week

- **Lean lamb, veal, or beef:** naturally raised with no hormones or antibiotics in small (3- to 4-ounce) portions no more than once or twice a month. (Note: Although prosciutto is forbidden, you can enjoy a little bit of Bundnerfleisch, air-dried beef, if from an excellent source.)

- **Small amounts of natural sweeteners:** maple syrup, honey, molasses, raw brown cane sugar, and stevia. (Note: No artificial sweeteners, such as aspartame, which is in almost all diet sodas, are allowed.)

- **Some nuts,** nut milks, nut butters, and seeds: cashews, pecans, macadamia nuts, coconut, sesame seeds, and pumpkin seeds

- **Lemon juice,** apple cider vinegar, balsamic vinegar, and other **mild vinegars**

- **Sea salt or Himalayan salt** in moderation, and most **herbs and spices**

- **Caffeine and alcohol** consumption is discouraged; one cup of coffee in the morning and one glass of wine in the evening, if you tolerate them

FOODS YOU *MUST NOT* EAT AT ANY TIME

- **All cow's milk,** including yogurt, cheeses, and ice cream. (Cholesterol and lacto-intolerance are not the issues here; allergy to cow protein is. Small amounts of organic butter or heavy cream are allowed occasionally.)

- **Pork.** It is dense in animal fat and high in sulfur, which thickens lymphatic fluids and is a toxic binder, because it attracts heavy metals and produces free radicals.

- **Shellfish.** Has a high risk of mercury, cadmium, and other heavy metals, arsenic, and toxins, and is one of the most common food allergens.

- **Bottom-feeding or large ocean fish,** such as swordfish, which are prone to high levels of mercury, PCBs, and other toxins

- **Processed foods,** which contain trans fats, preservatives, eggs, and dried milk

- **White flour**

- **Refined sugar**

- **Excessive sodium**

- **Soda,** whether sweetened with sugar or with artificial sweeteners, which in some ways are even more damaging

- **Commercial fruit juices,** especially orange juice; loaded with sugar and pesticides

- **Any genetically modified foods**

- **Many nuts,** especially hazelnuts, peanuts, and walnuts★

When you add up all the dos and don'ts, they translate to a diet that is most of all:

- Low in protein
- Alkaline in nature
- Free of food allergens, particularly cow dairy products
- High in omega-3 essential fatty acids
- With the correct balance of essential amino acids, especially from plant sources

Low Protein ·

It is the low-protein aspect of my diet that strikes some people as off-putting. Actually, I recommend the exact same number of grams as the United States government—40 to 60 grams a day; but most of my protein

---

★Nuts are problematic because they can cause severe allergic reactions. Different people are allergic to different nuts, and the prevalence even varies from country to country, probably because of childhood exposure. If you want to try adding certain forbidden nuts, such as almonds, to your diet and you know you don't have an overt histamine-based allergy to the nuts, you can introduce them with great care. For more information on these types of allergies and on how to introduce new foods, see Chapter 11. But always, a little bit is better than a lot.

WHEN DR. RAU SAYS NEVER

Giving up your favorite foods forever is not pleasing to most people. That's why so many of my patients like to say, "When Dr. Rau says 'never,' he means only once in a very great while." The truth is, as I've already mentioned, in many ways there is no cheating on my diet, because eating the wrong foods once in a very great while will not ordinarily impact your health.

But you have to weigh your risks. If you've cleaned out your system, which was in the past overly acidic and hyperproteinated, and you've been detoxified for months, a small steak or lamb chop or a sweet dessert will not do any damage. And if you are otherwise healthy and go on vacation and eat whatever you want for a week or two, you can always go back and detoxify again.

Your primary allergies, however, will always affect you, so keep that in mind. And some serious toxins, like heavy metals and PCBs, are permanently harmful in a way others are not. So when it comes to shellfish and large ocean fish, especially bottom feeders from the Atlantic, you may be wise to reconsider whether the risks are worth it or not.

Also, keep in mind the state of your health. If you are at present healthy and strong, you have more latitude. If you have a serious illness, your body deserves all the help and support it can get.

comes from plant sources that contain a very high amount of essential amino acids. Few people, however, adhere to the U.S. Department of Agriculture's Recommended Daily Allowance anyway.

Our entire lives, we are brainwashed into believing we require excessive amounts of meat and milk to grow strong and be smart and healthy. In terms of diet, we worry above all about not getting enough protein. The truth is, most people eat far more protein than their bodies can process on a cellular level. It is this overloading of protein that is the cause of most contemporary diseases. On my program, you get all the protein you need—mostly from vegetables and whole grains. (For more about protein requirements, see Chapter 5.)

Alkaline Balance

A healthy body is naturally slightly alkaline. This means the pH balance of the blood and other fluids is slightly alkaline rather than acidic. In a clinical setting, Darkfield microscopy shows acid–base shifts in the blood; but even at home, you can get some measure of your internal state with a simple color-coded urine test.

Metabolism of too much protein causes a buildup of acidity and ammonia, a toxic chemical, in the blood. It shifts the tissues to a slightly acidic composition, which has any number of biological consequences, especially for the ability of the red blood cells to pick up and transport oxygen to other cells. It also causes a slight congealing, or thickening, of the blood, lymph, and interstitial fluids, which promotes congestion and slows down metabolic processes. This has serious consequences for your immune system and leads to many diseases of the heart and circulatory system, such as arterial sclerosis and atherosclerosis.

You shift your body back into an alkaline balance by reducing protein consumption and eating a lot of fresh vegetables and fruits that are not too high in sugar.

Allergy Free

Cow dairy products are dense in amino acids not necessarily compatible with the human digestive tract. Cow's milk, yogurt, cheese, and, sadly, ice cream are major sources of many complications from food allergies. Often this allergy is confused with what people think is "lactose intolerance." Depending upon the individual, there may be any number of other food sensitivities. All of these cause congestion, inflammation, and impairment of the immune system. Weeding them out imparts a pleasing sensation of lightness in the gastrointestinal tract and greatly speeds up deep healing.

Omega-3s

These essential fatty acids are important to good health in many ways. They enhance cell metabolism, transmission of neural signals, and oxygenation of tissues, among other benefits. You cannot manufacture this nutrient; you obtain it by eating green, leafy vegetables and good fats, like flax seed oil and grape seed oil. It is also contained in oily fish, like sardines. While extra virgin olive oil does not contain omega-3s, if you have good intestinal flora, the bacteria will build omega-3s and the other essential fatty acids, omega-6s, for you.

Essential Amino Acids

Amino acids are the building blocks of protein. Your body must have access to all 20 amino acids in order to not only sustain life, but to thrive, grow, and heal. If you don't get all the amino acids needed from the food you eat, your body can actually manufacture 12 of them. However, 8 of the amino acids, called *essential amino acids*, cannot be reproduced and must be provided by your nutrition. Dr. Rau's Way prescribes foods whose proteins are well balanced in terms of the essential amino acids.

It's always easier to stick to a diet when you believe in its power. That's why I'd like you to understand the reasons behind the nutritional choices I've made. The following chapter details the science behind our epidemic of eating too much protein and why it leads to hyperacidity, which is terrible for your health. If you prefer, however, you can skip right to the Swiss Detox Diet.

CHAPTER FIVE

Putting Protein in Perspective

HYPERACIDITY AND DISEASE

As we've just discussed, Dr. Rau's Way is above all low in protein; alkaline in nature; free of known food allergies, especially cow dairy products; and rich in vegetables, fruits, and whole grains. Together, the recommended foods contribute a wide range of proteins plus the essential amino acids, vitamins, minerals, antioxidants, and omega-3 fatty acids your body needs. Before I get into the specifics of the diet plan, though, I want to address what is perhaps the most unconventional aspect of my program: *less protein*—much less protein—and the alkaline balance that accompanies it. Because the truth is, we don't really need very much protein. In fact, too much protein is counterproductive and damaging to your health.

Current U.S. government RDA guidelines suggest adults take in 15 to 20 percent of their daily calories from protein. For an average person, this translates to 50 to 60 grams of protein a day. This quantity was arrived at from several dietary studies done by major American institutions back in the 1980s, and it was published in the Surgeon General's Report, authored by C. Everett Koop, in 1988. Some organizations recommend a bit more than that. I recommend even less: 40 to 50 grams a day. (I'll tell you why a little later.)

Most Americans, however, end up eating 100 to 140 grams of protein every day—that's two and a half to three times as much as they need. For people on the Atkins and other low-carbohydrate diets and for hearty eaters who have meat—or chicken or fish—at each meal, the numbers can skyrocket even higher. The average American consumes more than 1½ pounds of meat, poultry, and seafood a day. And that doesn't even take into account other dense protein sources: eggs, cheese and other dairy products, and beans.

The belief that humans need eggs, steak, and quarts of milk every day derives from a laboratory experiment done with rats in the 1950s. As far

PROTEIN CONTENT OF COMMON FOODS

To give you an idea how fast protein can add up, here are a few numbers. Note that unless otherwise stated, these reflect 6-ounce portions. Think how often you are served an 8- or even 12-ounce portion, especially at restaurants.

CHICKEN BREAST, SKINLESS	45 grams
LEAN HAMBURGER	42 grams
GRILLED OR BROILED STEAK	38 grams
SALMON FILLET	34 grams
3 OUNCES CANNED TUNA	24 grams
1 CUP BEANS OR LENTILS	18 grams
1 CUP MILK	8 grams
1 CUP BROCCOLI	6 grams
1 EGG	6 grams
1 OUNCE CHEESE	4–7 grams
1 TABLESPOON PEANUT BUTTER	4 grams
1 CUP RICE	4 grams

back as 1988, however, studies done by the American Association of Dieticians (AAD) proved that in this respect, rats are different from humans. (Should we be surprised?)

First, these studies showed our protein requirements are much more modest than a rodent's. They also demonstrated that when humans are fed a meatless diet that includes any combination of vegetables eaten with either wheat or rice, there is absolutely no evidence of lack of protein in the blood. Indeed, we know of many societies that have thrived with absolutely no meat at all in their diets. Some vegetarian cultures are famous for their longevity.

The fact is, even if you get no meat in your diet, you almost assuredly will get enough protein from other sources not only to survive, but to thrive. Proteins are present in almost all foods. It's the quality rather than the quantity that counts. But somehow, this information was never publicized. Advertising and lobbying from the beef and dairy industry as well as the fact that meat and fat taste so good to many people somehow distracted the American public and perpetuated the protein myth.

Consequently, no one worries about getting enough carbohydrates. No one worries about getting enough fat and essential fatty acids. But many people mistakenly worry about getting enough protein. Quite the opposite is true: Most people should worry about getting *too much* protein.

There are no documented cases of protein deficiency from diet in the United States. Clinical protein deficiency, a disease called kwashiorkor, with a distinctive wasting look and loss of pigmentation, exists almost exclusively in extremely poor and war-devastated areas where people are literally starving to death. Or where they don't get enough of the *essential amino acids.*

The Importance of Amino Acids

Proteins are often referred to as the building blocks of your body. That's because proteins drive every hormonal and metabolic function in your body, and every cell is maintained by and new cells built from different proteins. Of course, not all cells are alike. Under a microscope, your lung cells, for example, look different from your skin cells; red blood cells look different from white bloods cells. That's because proteins in turn are constructed from different amino acids arranged in varying configurations. So it's more accurate, and practical from a nutritional point of view, to think about our dietary needs in terms of individual amino acids.

All protein is made up of amino acids; 20 of these are encoded by our DNA. We get these from different foods, which vary in their amino acid composition. For some time, it was believed that people needed to combine proteins at every meal—for example, corn, rice, and beans, which together contain all the amino acids, thus making a "complete" protein. This has been disproved in many major studies. Even the most conservative dietician today will allow that you do not need to eat complementary proteins at every meal or even every day. You can eat a variety of foods during the week or over several weeks. After digestion, your liver mixes and matches to come up with just the right blend of amino acids necessary to build the proteins your body signals it needs.

Your Body Manufactures Proteins

In addition, your body can make the proteins it needs. Recent scientific studies have shown that among its many functions, the liver actually synthesizes new amino acids from old and damaged proteins that are being discarded. That's why Dr. Rau's Way recommends you eat only 40 to 50 grams of protein a day; no more is needed. If a part of your body calls for an amino

THE AMINO ACIDS—
ESSENTIAL AND NONESSENTIAL

ESSENTIAL AMINO ACIDS
    isoleucine, leucine, lysine, methionine, phenylalanine, threonine, tryptophan, valine

NONESSENTIAL AMINO ACIDS
    alanine, arginine, asparagine, aspartic acid, cysteine, glutamic acid, glutamine, glycine, histidine, proline, serine, tyrosine

acid not readily available from food, the liver can make it up, like an apothecary mixing a tonic from the many ingredients he or she has on hand.

Even if you ate almost no protein, you could get most of what you needed from your own body for months, *except* for the eight amino acids your body cannot construct. These vital building blocks, which must be acquired through food, are called the *essential amino acids*. For proper optimization and use of proteins to maintain health and build and repair cells, you must ingest these essential amino acids, because your body cannot produce them from scratch.

Essential amino acid requirements are not large. Each day, all you need is a maximum of 15 to 20 grams. Conceptually, you could think of the essential amino acids as really strong glue. You only need a little bit compared to the rest of the amino acids, but they are vital to the strength of the structure, critical for your health. What is important, then, is not just *how much* protein, but *what kind* of protein. And there are much better sources of high-quality protein than meat. My diet prescribes meals containing foods like peas, corn, beans, avocados, soy products, chestnuts, and quinoa, which are properly balanced in proteins and rich in these essential amino acids. So assuming you are getting enough of the essential amino acids, much of the remaining protein is not only superfluous, but counterproductive.

Too Much Protein Is Damaging

What happens to the extra protein you don't use? Your liver acts as the trash collector, "digesting" as much as it can, which produces ammonia, a substance toxic to humans. Normally, the liver converts this ammonia to urea and passes it off to the kidneys, which dispose of it in urine. Too much protein actually puts a strain on the kidneys. For every 50 grams of protein digested, your body must contribute 3 cups of water to dilute the resulting uric acid that is excreted. That's why you urinate frequently after eating meat.

As a comparison, metabolizing an equal amount of fat or carbohydrates consumes less than ½ cup of water. Unless you are careful to drink enough water, digesting too much protein can cause dehydration, which stresses the kidneys. Excess protein coupled with the dehydration it causes can lead to urinary tract infections and is a major cause of painful kidney stones.

When there is so much protein being processed that the system cannot handle it all, ammonia backs up into the blood, leading to both hyperacidity and a toxicity so great that if it continued, a person could collapse and eventually die. Who would think you could be poisoned by what you ate? Yet recently, hospitals have been seeing such cases associated with people who have followed high-protein/low-carbohydrate diets for a long time.

Too much protein—like too much of many good things—actually does more harm than good. In fact, I believe that *hyperproteinemia*—that is, too much protein in the blood—is one of the main causes of a host of our most dreaded diseases: especially heart disease and cancer. With Americans eating upward of three and four times the amount of protein they need, we shouldn't be surprised when we see that rates of obesity, hypertension, and diabetes are skyrocketing—even in children.

Here's a simpler way to think about hyperproteinemia. We all know, from folktales if from nowhere else, that when it comes to survival, materials make a big difference. In "The Three Little Pigs," the Big Bad Wolf had no trouble blowing down houses made of straw and of sticks. But the house built of bricks resisted his most furious blows. He huffed and he puffed, but he got nowhere.

Just like the Big Bad Wolf, the great winds of hurricanes and tornadoes take out flimsy mobile homes first. That's why monuments and public buildings designed to last are constructed from strong materials: stone and brick. Getting the construction of a sturdy house completed, however, can be quite a task, and building takes time. You have to calculate all your needs, round up your supplies, make sure you have a design that is both elegant and sound, and then hire workmen to build the structure—not to speak of supervising them and tinkering with changes as you go along.

Most importantly, you must spend the time and effort necessary to be sure your house has an excellent foundation. Without that base, the entire structure might fall down. Of course, you could put up a prefab house overnight or tow a mobile home into place, but neither would have the strength of a house built of bricks and would not last nearly as long.

Think of the *nonessential* amino acids that make up proteins as the bricks that form the building blocks of your house, and the *essential* amino acids as the mortar, or cement. You have your plans, and your architect knows a wonderfully skilled builder who will build the walls. They have found an excellent source for fine, high-quality bricks. Sounds like you are all set to begin construction.

On day one, the supplier drops off a pallet of bricks and some bags of mortar mix. The bricklayer gets to work. At first, he's a little slow, because he is new to the job; and anyway, the base is the thickest part of the wall. But all goes well, and by the end of the day, he's used up all the bricks. However, there are a couple of bags of mortar mix left over.

The architect is watching, and thinks, "Why not get more bricks so the bricklayer can work faster?" Plus the supplier will give him a discount if he buys more bricks at once. So on day two, the supplier delivers two pallets of bricks. The bricklayer works as fast as he can, but by the end of the day, he runs out of mortar mix, so he can get through only one and a half pallets. The remainder of the bricks are just lying around in the way. He knows he has another delivery coming in the morning, so he instructs his assistant to pile up the unused bricks. They'll use them later.

The next day, the bricklayer works as fast as he can, but he's a little inconvenienced by the piles of extra bricks he has to work around. So he and his assistant take time off and move the piles behind the house. Much less wall goes up than the day before. The bricklayer tries to convince the architect to reduce the order, but the architect thinks it is good to have extra bricks at such a good price. If there are a lot left over, he will design an arboretum to go behind the house.

Each day, too many bricks arrive, and they pile up both in front of and behind the house. Soon, there are so many bricks lying around and the piles are so high, the bricklayer has trouble working around them. He and his assistant start spending more time moving the bricks around than building the walls. His productivity suffers greatly, and the quality of his work slides way downhill. In addition, to try and save some time, he even instructs his assistant to use a thinner layer of mortar.

Finally, the piles are so high, work comes to a standstill. There's nothing the bricklayer can do to get rid of all those bricks. The pile behind the house is bigger than the beautiful foundation walls he has constructed. Suddenly a squall with high gusts of wind passes through. That huge pile of bricks in back starts swaying and as the bricklayer watches in horror, it comes crashing down on the house, destroying the beautiful foundation wall he had put so much effort into building.

Why did the pile of bricks come crashing down even though they were so heavy? *Because there was no mortar holding them together for strength.* It had no structural integrity. And why did the foundation wall of the house collapse? *Partly because it was overpowered by the weight of the bricks and partly because it was weakened by not having enough mortar.*

Metaphorically, that's what happens when there is too much protein in your body. And not only does your body have to deal with the proteins you ingest, it also has to dispose of old, degraded proteins from cells that have finished their life span. The ones that die off must be disposed of somehow. There are mechanisms in the body, some of which have only recently become well understood, that essentially digest the protein walls of these now-useless cells and revert them to their component parts—think of a garbage disposal grinding up peelings.

Waste materials are flushed out through the liver and kidneys, but many of the valuable molecules are reused, combined in new ways to make new amino acids that can, in turn, be used to construct many of the valuable proteins the body requires. But to make usable new proteins, the liver has to have enough essential amino acids to act as binder. If the essential amino acids are available to use as mortar, these bits of degraded amino acids can be rebuilt into strong new proteins.

What the liver cannot dispose of must be stored in some way. Excess degraded amino acids get backed up in the blood and lymph systems and in the interstitial fluids, causing congestion and hyperacidity. This is a leading cause of many chronic degenerative and inflammatory illnesses.

Less Protein for Better Health

Your body takes nutrients in and processes and changes them so they can be used as needed. What's left over, the waste products, are eliminated through urine, stool, sweat, and breath.

As described, we take proteins in, and we release proteins. At the same time, the human being is a dynamic system, not a marble statue that doesn't change. Not only are the proteins changed when you eat them, *you* are changed. Protein metabolism produces acid. Remember, to ward off disease and heal yourself, to look and feel as good as possible, your internal environment must be slightly alkaline. Too much protein, like too much nitrogen in the soil, will simply lead to rot.

Big problems arise not because there is too little protein in the diet, but too much. Many metabolic weaknesses and chronic diseases arise when so many amino acids are squeezed into the body that they cannot be eliminated properly. Like any chemical factory, the liver can do only so much work in any given day. If you overload the recycling bin, as it were, you're going to run into trouble. Another way to think of it is like this:

All cellular metabolism, the "breathing" that all living cells must do, produces by-products, like ash from a wood fire. When you start a fire, it produces light and warmth. At first, it may be a little weak, but once the wood catches, the fire becomes hot and gives off good light, too. As it burns, a chemical change takes place as energy is released from the wood. The hard wood is transformed into powdery ash, which falls to the floor of the stove.

You decide you want the fire to burn hotter, so you add more wood. At first, this plan works well. But if you keep adding wood and don't clean out the ashes from the bottom, the lack of oxygen will begin to smother the fire. What was once a bright, very efficient flame will dim and become less effective.

So it is with your body. When we eat not only too much protein, but also too much sugar and toxic substances that cannot be reused, these substances are eliminated through urine, stool, sweat, and breath. Like too much wood in the fire, though, if we continue to take in too many proteins and toxic products, our ability to recycle them diminishes along with our ability to eliminate them.

When we cannot properly eliminate excess proteins, these toxins become stored throughout the body, largely in the form of free radicals, which are extremely dangerous, because they have open bonds and can form other chemicals, many of them carcinogenic. When there's no free eliminatory flow, these free radicals get stuck within the cells, and cell function weakens or decreases.

Excess proteins are also forced into the blood vessels, connective tissue, and lymph, causing what Swiss biological medicine calls "deposit diseases": obesity, hypertension, and coronary heart disease, among others. The more free radicals and degraded proteins stuck inside the cells, the poorer the function of those cells.

This is why the Swiss Detox Diet avoids as much protein as possible, especially during the first week. There is much cleanup and recycling work to do. The goal is to open up the pathways and allow as many old proteins and toxins as possible to be flushed out.

Because it is in the storage and metabolizing of excess protein that the body runs into trouble, my nutritional plan focuses on a wide variety of plant sources, like vegetables and whole grains, for most of the amino acids you need, with small amounts of chicken and fish as well as moderate amounts of other protein-rich foods, such as beans, tofu, eggs, and dairy. Like the bricklayer, your body can only process about 40 grams of protein a day; the rest becomes waste.

At the same time, while protein intake is greatly diminished, my diet ensures that you get at least 12 to 15 grams of essential amino acids each day. This encourages the liver to recycle old proteins and use them to build fresh new cells. Most people who have vague symptoms or chronic systemic problems traditional medicine has not been effective at treating, and especially people who are truly sick, are hyperproteinized. They cannot constructively use all the old proteins backed up in their system.

The only way to get rid of this overflow is with the essential amino acids, which enable the liver to use nonessential amino acids from the old proteins to build new, vital cells, thus lightening the toxic load. Sometimes this takes weeks, sometimes months, and sometimes even years.

The Dangers of Hyperacidity

Another problem caused by the overconsumption of protein is hyperacidity. What does this mean? Think what happens when you stir lemon juice or vinegar into milk: it curdles. When your internal environment is acidic, this same thickening happens to your blood, your lymphatic fluids, and the fluids that flow in the tiny spaces between your cells, called the interstitial fluids. These tiny spaces are very important, because it is there that the cells, such as neurons and components of the immune system, communicate with each other.

When the body is hyperacidic and these fluids thicken, many vital processes slow down: cell respiration—how a cell uses oxygen and "breathes"—nerve impulses, immune responses, and production of important regulatory enzymes and hormones. In the midst of this congestion, signals slow down, toxins collect, and cell metabolism becomes sluggish. Cellular nutrition actually decreases, and nutrients cannot reach the cells. In spite of the excess of proteins, the cells themselves are forced into a "starving" situation. This results in early aging.

At the same time, the body responds to the acidic environment by drawing out calcium and other minerals from the bones and connective tissues to buffer the acid. The Women's Health Initiative, a 15-year study of close to 162,000 women sponsored by the National Institutes of Health, found that over a 12-year period, women who consumed more than 95 grams of protein daily had a 20 percent greater chance of breaking a wrist than women who took in less than 68 grams a day.

We see that over the long term, hyperproteinated, hyperacidic patients develop all the degenerative diseases. These include many of the major problems of Western civilization. It's interesting to wonder why Americans, in particular, are encouraged to eat so much meat and dairy products.

Worst of all, in a hyperacidic environment, eventually the microorganisms, the symbionts we learned about in Chapter 1, which contribute to our vitality in their healthy state, are transmuted into a pathological state, which allows illness to develop.

An acidic internal environment can arise not only from too much protein but also from too much sugar in the diet. So there are any number of reasons for avoiding sugar. It causes spikes and then deep drops in blood sugar, which reduces energy, focus, and performance. Too much sugar in the blood can lead to type 2 diabetes. White sugar is processed with arsenic, a poison. And sugar metabolism leads to acidity of the internal environment.

When trying to avoid sugar, look not only at your sugar bowl, but also at the labels of many processed foods. There are hidden sugars all over the place: high-fructose corn syrup, maltose, and dextrose are all sugars of one sort or another. Even fructose, which is fruit sugar, can be damaging if

SOME EFFECTS OF LONG-TERM HYPERACIDITY

When cells are essentially "strangled" by long-term hyperacidity, caused by too much protein and sugar in the diet, physical consequences vary, depending upon where your body is most vulnerable. The most common problems that result are:

- Hypertension, or high blood pressure
- Decrease in microcirculation, which leads to coronary heart diseases, arterial sclerosis, and memory problems
- Degenerative joint diseases, such as osteoarthritis
- Osteoporosis
- Disc problems, which result in back pain
- All kinds of cancer
- Impaired glandular function
- Stomach and intestinal problems
- Insomnia

amounts in the diet are too high. Also, keep in mind that refined carbohydrates, like white flour, end up processing into simple sugars in the body as well.

Given that heart disease is the leading cause of death in America, it is particularly interesting to understand the relationship between blood acidity and heart disease. A disturbance of the body's healthy alkaline balance affects the arteries in several ways. First of all, when blood becomes acidic, the electrical charge on the outside of the red blood cells actually alters, causing them to stick together like magnets. We saw this in the picture of rouleaux on page 32. When the blood cells stick together like this, they have a much higher chance of forming clots, which can lead to strokes.

Hyperacidity also contributes to atherosclerosis, or hardening of the arteries. Contrary to popular belief, cholesterol is not the primary problem with plaque in the arteries; it's the hyperacidity and mineral shifts in the tissues. When the body starts to become acidic, calcium and other minerals are drawn out of the bones and the magnesium from the cartilage into the connective tissues and interstitial spaces and even arteries in an effort to buffer, or neutralize, the acid. When these minerals that are drawn out react with cholesterol that is naturally in the blood, calcified deposits form, which is how atherosclerosis develops. If you follow my nutritional plan over the long term, cholesterol levels of most people will normalize themselves without any need for drugs.

So we see that it is not cholesterol, but too much dietary protein that leads to a host of chronic degenerative, inflammatory, and autoimmune diseases: cancer, atherosclerosis, arterial sclerosis, heart disease, stroke, arthritis, type 2 diabetes, and mainly osteoporosis. They all arise from different pathways, but one main factor contributes to each: too much protein in the diet.

A basic understanding of the reasons for all the dietary choices I make will help you feel comfortable with what at first glance might seem like an unconventional nutritional program. Knowledge will also make it easier to stay on the right path, even over time. For eating well is the best thing you can do for your health.

What is different about Dr. Rau's Way is that, while my dietary plan not only eliminates red meat and allows only a very modest amount of chicken and fish, it also doesn't pad your diet with dairy products, eggs, beans, or tofu to compensate. It simply calls for less protein—period! One of the primary reasons for this is to counteract acidity and place the body in a benign alkaline balance.

That's why Dr. Rau's Way gives you a blueprint for nutrition that will forge a robust, health-inducing constitution, allowing just enough of the proteins you need and all the essential amino acids to do the job well. If we want our bodies to last long and serve us well, to protect us from ill-

CONSEQUENCES OF HYPERACIDITY
FROM PROTEIN OVERLOAD

Several things happen when the internal environment becomes acidic and
bodily fluids thicken:

- Congestion of the blood leads to clots, which can cause stroke and a
  buildup of plaque.

- Red blood cells clump together, which means they have less surface
  area and are less efficient. Because these are the cells that carry oxygen to all your tissues, this reduces cell metabolism, slows healing,
  and leads to weight gain.

- In an effort to buffer acidity, calcium and other minerals are leached
  from the bones, causing osteoporosis and compromising the structural integrity of the bone. When this excess calcium in the blood en-
  counters cholesterol deposits in the arteries, it causes them to
  harden, producing atherosclerosis, or hardening of the arteries.

- This same leaching of minerals, especially magnesium, from cartilage brings on osteoarthritis.

- When the lymph and interstitial fluids thicken, cells cannot communicate as efficiently with each other, and the entire immune system is
  suppressed.

- Conduction of nerve impulses slows down in the congested environment, much like light in a pea-soup fog.

- The tiny microorganisms in the blood that we call bionts mutate into
  pathological states, reducing vitality and instigating disease.

HOW HYPERACIDITY EXPRESSES ITSELF
IN THE ORGANS

Hyperacidity in the blood also causes a host of problems in the organs and other tissues. Depending on the organ, the disturbance will be expressed in different ways:

KIDNEY/BLADDER . . . . Cystitis, prostate enlargement, kidney stones, yeast infections in women

STOMACH . . . . Acid reflux, ulcers

SKIN . . . . Excess sweating, rashes, swelling, eczema

INTESTINES . . . . Colitis, bowel irregularity

LUNGS . . . . Asthma, recurrent bronchitis

JOINTS . . . . Arthritis, myalgia

NEUROLOGICAL SYSTEM . . . . Depression, decreased alertness, fatigue

ness and ward off degeneration caused by age, they must be constructed properly from the right materials.

But before you build upon all you've learned, you must dig out your foundation. To remedy an existing acidic internal environmental and to remove other factors that are impeding your path to healing, you must first clean out your system before any adjustments to your health can take hold. That's why my Swiss Detox Diet comes first.

CHAPTER SIX

The Swiss Detox Diet

PUTTING YOUR BODY BACK IN BALANCE

So many of my patients have benefited from this extremely effective diet that it's hard to know where to begin. What's particularly of note is that it is a nutritional program that is excellent for almost everyone. The Paracelsus Clinic's experience with thousands of patients (30,000 on record) has proven that it works well for an exceptionally wide variety of problems.

Of course, it benefits those who are healthy and wish to remain so and those who want to strengthen themselves and feel even better. It is rejuvenating for anyone who is run-down or feels old before his time. But it has a truly amazing effect on people with undefined intestinal, abdominal, mental, and rheumatic ailments (joint and connective tissue diseases) as well as for those suffering from allergies, arthritis, and cardiovascular problems. We have healed more than two-thirds of our colitis patients on this diet alone. It has tremendous value as well for those with vague diagnoses, mild metabolic imbalances, general malaise, depression, and familial genetic propensities for illnesses they'd like to avoid. And the Swiss Detox Diet is of immense value as yet another tool in helping patients who suffer from a range of serious chronic inflammatory and degenerative diseases.

PHYSICAL BENEFITS OF THE SWISS DETOX DIET

In as little as three weeks, you can profit from this carefully prescribed, easy-to-follow diet in the following ways:

- Increased mental alertness
- Improved sexual function
- Deeper, more restful sleep
- Reduced allergies, which means fewer headaches and sinus problems
- Greater energy and vitality, with even blood sugar levels throughout the day
- Reduced susceptibility to infections

The Swiss Detox Diet is an important part of our treatment of chronic fatigue, multiple sclerosis, and fibromyalgia. And it provides the appropriate nutrition for all chronic autoimmune and cancer patients, as well. Note: The only exceptions for whom this diet must be altered are patients with a genetically fixed gluten allergy—that is, celiac disease—and those who have a severe fructose intolerance. Also, pregnant and nursing women should skip the Swiss Detox Diet and go straight to the Maintenance Diet for Life.

The reason this nutritional program is so helpful to so many is that it provides the fertile soil, as it were, needed to nourish the internal environment, preparing you for deep healing. Primarily, it is a diet of regulation. By that I mean it strengthens your body and balances the up-building and degenerative forces on a number of different fronts. Because it detoxifies your body for three weeks, it has a powerful effect. The Swiss Detox Diet:

- Detoxifies the body
- De-acidifies the internal environment
- Develops proper intestinal flora

By so doing, it:

- Regulates metabolism
- Encourages healing
- Rebuilds the immune system
- Restores the health of major organs

How does it accomplish so much? For one thing, the Swiss Detox Diet keeps digging away at your toxic load, literally digesting it and eliminating it from your body. You've spent your entire life accumulating a wide range of what we call disturbances, or toxic foci. It should be no surprise that it can take weeks—if not years—to repair the damage. Some serious problems, of course, require further treatment at a biological medicine center. But this is the best way to begin.

My diet alkalizes your body and de-acidifies your blood and internal organs, which has a tremendously energizing effect on your metabolism. If you are overweight, you will see the pounds melt away; if you are in need of nutrition, you will be pleased with your weight gain. After as little as 10 days, most everyone feels deeply energized.

The composition of foods chosen for detox are such that metabolism actually increases. All hormones—ovarian, thyroid, melatonin, and so on—stay the same, while pituitary hormones remain stable and, in some cases, even increase. At the same time, gallbladder and liver counts decrease; bile is loosened, and flow increases enormously. For many people with high cholesterol levels, counts often return to normal levels within one to three weeks.

Technically speaking, cholesterol is lowered because it gets processed along natural pathways into progesterone in women or into DHEA/ testosterone in men. Therefore, sex hormones often increase on this nutritional program, noticeably in some men with problems like erectile dysfunction.

One distinctive feature of the diet is the palette of ingredients it uses. These are not chosen arbitrarily or for their low caloric or fat content, but because with these foods we effectively eliminate *90 percent* of common adult food allergies. Because the diet is followed for a full three weeks, your entire immune system is given a chance to turn over completely, as we explained earlier. Individual results will vary, of course, depending upon your particular food intolerances—and everyone has them, whether you know it or not.

By the end of the three weeks, many troubling symptoms you thought were yours forever will suddenly disappear. These include headaches, sinus infections, rashes, muscle and joint aches, lethargy, inability to focus, and depression. Healing will speed up. You will feel stronger and lighter. You may well find yourself calmer than you have been in years. Your blood sugar level will remain level all day. You will sleep well, going to bed earlier at night, and waking up fully rested.

Three weeks is an important milestone; but if you are obese or especially if you are seriously ill, I urge you to repeat the program for six or even nine weeks. This extra time will be of enormous benefit; it offers the best opportunity to heal some serious chronic diseases at a deep cellular level. And given the delicious menus designed for you, you may well find the diet more of a pleasure than a chore.

To allow for variety, each day's meal plan gives you an enticing choice of salads and vegetables. For convenience, many of the salads can be made in advance and eaten two or three days in a row. Shredded raw and lightly steamed vegetables form the bedrock of this diet. The first week is completely vegan—mostly fresh vegetables with small amounts of fruit and very little grain, with a minimum of gluten. In the second and third weeks, very modest portions of goat and sheep cheese, legumes, and more whole grains are included as well as natural sweeteners.

To make the diet palatable, the menus call for delicious recipes, most of which were developed specifically for this book. They are simple and will make sure you get the proper nutrition you need. However, if you would prefer to follow the Swiss Detox Diet with virtually no cooking at all, you can design your own menus at lunch and dinner as long as you restrict yourself solely to Dr. Rau's Alkaline Soup and shredded raw and lightly steamed green vegetables. If you do so, make sure you are careful to dress the vegetables with at least 1 tablespoon fresh lemon juice and extra virgin olive oil at each meal and to sprinkle sunflower seeds, pumpkin seeds, or flax seeds over your salads. If you choose this freeform diet, be sure to include small amounts of goat and sheep cheese or yogurt and spelt bread during weeks two and three. When in doubt, refer to the daily diets for amounts.

If a particular vegetable on any menu called for is unavailable, you may substitute any of the other vegetables listed in the diet. Likewise, if you don't feel like making one of the prepared salads, you can always substitute a simple shredded raw vegetable, dressed with fresh lemon juice and extra virgin olive oil. And if you don't like variety and wish to eat the same breakfast every day, pick your favorite. Here are a few dos and don'ts that will make the diet easier to follow:

- At lunch you should have both raw and cooked vegetables, but at night you should eat cooked vegetables only.

- No fruit should be eaten after 4:00 in the afternoon. It ferments in the gut at night, stressing the liver.

- Do not skip midmorning and afternoon snacks. They are crucial to maintaining blood sugar levels and warding off hunger.

- You *must* drink at least 3 liters of herb tea and purified water a day.

- Begin your day with ½ measuring spoon of Pleo Alkala (spoon provided with package) or other alkalizing powder, such as bicarbonate of soda, dissolved in an 8-ounce glass of warm water.

- Each morning should begin with a cup of broth of Dr. Rau's Alkaline Soup.

A Meal Plan for Total Detox

On this excellent diet, you will find that you enjoy a satisfying—and alkalizing—breakfast; a substantial lunch, which is your largest meal of the day; and a light supper. Vegetables make up by far the bulk of the diet. No coffee, caffeinated beverages, sugar, meat, wheat products, cow dairy products, or alcohol is allowed. Stay away from decaf tea and coffee, which still contain small amounts of caffeine. Restrict yourself to herbal teas and my alkaline broth for this period of cleansing. Table salt, sodium chloride, is absolutely prohibited; in fact, at no stage of my plan should you use this salt. However, you may use modest amounts of naturally evaporated sea salt or mined Himalayan salt.

Stock up on organic vegetables, lemons, and grapefruits. Follow the program exactly as indicated. Eat slowly and chew your food extremely well. In addition to the menus detailed here, you must drink 2 to 3 liters of pure, noncarbonated mineral water and herbal tea each day. Water should be taken after—not during—meals. Drinking too much water with meals can dilute the stomach acids and impede proper digestion.

Remember that to accomplish the goals of this excellent nutritional program, you must follow it as designed. Perhaps you are used to nothing but coffee in the morning or just a bite of toast. Well, perhaps that's part of the reason your body is rebelling now. Whatever your state of illness or health, this diet has been very carefully calculated. You must eat everything, even if you think you are full; and if you are hungry, which would be unusual, simply have some extra steamed leafy greens. Because of the large amounts of vegetables and fluids called for, though, hunger is rarely an issue.

WEEK ONE

Breakfast

- Cup **or** small bowl of broth only (no vegetables) from Dr. Rau's Alkaline Soup (page 152)

- 4 ounces (½ cup) fresh grapefruit juice, preferably Ruby Red, **or** ½ grapefruit

- 1 tablespoon pure flax seed oil

- ¼ cup steel-cut oats cooked in 1 cup water with 1 date until very soft, about 15 minutes; no other sweetener

- 1 small apple (Note: Apple is good diced and eaten with oatmeal) **or** ½ avocado, dressed with 1 tablespoon freshly squeezed lemon juice and 1 teaspoon extra virgin olive oil

- 1 cup decaffeinated green tea **or** herb tea

Midmorning Snack

- ½ apple **or** 1 small carrot

Lunch

- SALAD PLATE: Your choice of shredded raw vegetables dressed with lemon juice and extra virgin olive oil **or** ⅓ cup Shredded Beet and Carrot Salad (page 218); ⅓ cup shredded zucchini tossed with 1½ teaspoons fresh lemon juice and 1 teaspoon extra virgin olive oil; ½ cup Asian Sesame Slaw (page 219)

- STEAMED VEGETABLE PLATE: Broccoli florets, sliced carrots, and 1 small Yukon gold potato, sliced, all lightly steamed; do not overcook. May splash with 2 teaspoons each lemon juice **or** balsamic vinegar and extra virgin olive oil **or** sunflower oil. Sprinkle with 1 tablespoon sunflower seeds.

NOTES FOR THE COOK

- All fruits and vegetables should be both fresh and organic.

- Water used for drinking and cooking should be noncarbonated and nonchlorinated. Bottled purified or spring water is recommended.

- Grated raw vegetables are an important part of the program, so pull out the shredding disk of your food processor or use the large holes on a box grater.

- If you don't own a good stainless-steel steamer, it is well worth the investment since you will eat plenty of steamed vegetable in every stage of Dr. Rau's Way. In fact, once you discover how delicious organic vegetables taste when lightly steamed, you will stop thinking of them as diet food and begin looking forward to them.

- No table salt—sodium chloride with chemicals—ever! Choose naturally evaporated sea salt or Himalayan salt.

Midafternoon Snack

- ½ avocado, 6 cucumber sticks, or ½ apple

Supper

- 4 ounces (½ cup) fresh carrot **or** other vegetable juice

- Bowl of Dr. Rau's Alkaline Soup, including ½ cup diced vegetables from the soup

- ½ cup (after cooking) Olive Oil–Steamed Spinach (page 252)

- ½ cup steamed broccoli florets

- Cup of herb tea, such as peppermint

WEEK ONE | DAY 2

Breakfast

- Same as Day 1

Midmorning Snack

- Same as Day 1

Lunch

- SALAD PLATE: Your choice of shredded raw vegetables dressed with lemon juice and extra virgin olive oil **or** 1 cup shredded Romaine lettuce, 1 medium carrot, shredded, 2 tablespoons cooked chickpeas, and 2 tablespoons very thinly sliced red bell pepper, tossed with 1 tablespoon each fresh lemon juice and extra virgin olive oil

- STEAMED ORGANIC VEGETABLE PLATE: Cauliflower florets, green beans, and 1 small sweet potato, lightly steamed; do not overcook. May splash with 2 teaspoons each lemon juice **or** balsamic vinegar and extra virgin olive oil **or** sunflower oil. Sprinkle with 1 tablespoon pumpkin seeds.

Midafternoon Snack

- Same as Day 1

Supper

- 4 ounces (½ cup) fresh beet **or** other vegetable juice

- Bowl of Dr. Rau's Alkaline Soup, including ½ cup diced vegetables from the soup

- 1 cup steamed broccoli florets plus ½ cup steamed sliced potatoes, dressed with fresh lemon juice and extra virgin olive oil

- Cup of herb tea

Breakfast

- Same as Day 1

Midmorning Snack

- Same as Day 1

Lunch

- SALAD PLATE: Your choice of shredded raw vegetables dressed with lemon juice and extra virgin olive oil **or** ½ cup Swiss Potato Salad (page 224), made with no leek; ½ cup (loosely packed) alfalfa sprouts; ⅓ cup Shredded Beet and Carrot Salad

- STEAMED VEGETABLE PLATE: Swiss chard, zucchini slices, and sliced peeled kohlrabi **or** celery root lightly steamed; do not overcook. May splash with 2 teaspoons each lemon juice **or** balsamic vinegar and extra virgin olive oil **or** sunflower oil. Serve with 2 tablespoons cooked **or** sprouted lentils.

Midafternoon Snack

- Same as Day 1

Supper

- 4 ounces (½ cup) fresh carrot **or** other vegetable juice

- Bowl of Dr. Rau's Alkaline Soup, including ½ cup diced vegetables from the soup

- ½ cup diced butternut squash and 1 cup loosely packed baby spinach leaves, steamed and tossed with balsamic vinegar and extra virgin olive oil

- Cup of herb tea

Breakfast

- Same as Day 1

Midmorning Snack

- Same as Day 1

Lunch

- SALAD PLATE: Your choice of shredded raw vegetables dressed with lemon juice and olive oil **or** 1 cup baby spinach leaves; 1 medium carrot, peeled and shredded; ½ cup bean sprouts; and ⅓ cup shredded cucumber tossed with 1 tablespoon each fresh lemon juice and extra virgin olive oil. Sprinkle with 2 teaspoons flax seeds.

- STEAMED VEGETABLE PLATE: Cut-up asparagus **or** broccoli, carrot slices, and 1 small potato, sliced and lightly steamed; do not overcook. May splash with 2 teaspoons each lemon juice **or** balsamic vinegar and extra virgin olive oil **or** sunflower oil.

Midafternoon Snack

- Same as Day 1

Supper

- 4 ounces (½ cup) fresh beet **or** other vegetable juice
- Bowl of Dr. Rau's Alkaline Soup, including ½ cup diced vegetables from the soup
- 1 globe artichoke, steamed and served with fresh lemon juice blended with extra virgin olive oil and a pinch of sea salt for dipping
- If you need it: 1 small sweet potato, baked and mashed with 1 teaspoon sunflower oil
- Cup of herb tea

WEEK ONE | DAY 5

Breakfast

- Same as Day 1

Midmorning Snack

- Same as Day 1

Lunch

- SALAD PLATE: Your choice of shredded raw vegetables dressed with lemon juice and olive oil **or** ½ cup raw **or** lightly steamed cauliflower florets, ¼ cup shredded carrot, and ¼ cup shredded zucchini **or** cucumber, and arugula leaves tossed with 2 teaspoons each lemon juice **or** balsamic vinegar and 2 teaspoons extra virgin olive oil **or** sunflower oil

- STEAMED VEGETABLE PLATE: Halved Brussels sprouts **or** shredded cabbage, ½ cup sliced garnet yam **or** sweet potato, Swiss chard lightly steamed; do not overcook. Also, ¼ cup Spiced Steamed Chickpeas (page 191), made with no salt

Midafternoon Snack

- Same as Day 1

Supper

- 4-ounce glass (½ cup) fresh carrot **or** other vegetable juice

- Bowl of Dr. Rau's Alkaline Soup, including ½ cup diced vegetables from the soup

- 1 cup steamed broccoli florets plus 1 small potato, dressed with fresh lemon juice and extra virgin olive oil

- Cup of herb tea

WEEK ONE | DAY 6

Breakfast

- Same as Day 1

Midmorning Snack

- Same as Day 1

Lunch

- May repeat any day, except Day 5

Midafternoon Snack

- Same as Day 1

Supper

- Same as Day 1, 3, **or** 4

WEEK ONE | DAY 7

Breakfast

- Same as Day 1

Midmorning Snack

- Same as Day 1

Lunch

- May repeat any day, except Day 6

Midafternoon Snack

- Same as Day 1

Supper

■ Same as Day 1, 3, **or** 4

WEEK TWO

While maintaining an alkaline balance and continuing to restrict food allergens, the menus for week two gradually incorporate small amounts of whole grains and goat and sheep dairy to vary your diet and broaden your nutritional base. Whenever you have salad, know that you can always embellish it with a light sprinkling of sunflower seeds, pumpkin seeds, or flax seeds.

Don't forget to continue to drink copious amounts (at least 3 liters) of purified water, unsweetened herb tea, and my alkalizing broth. Begin your day with a glass of warm water and ½ measuring spoon of Alkala or other alkalizing powder, such as bicarbonate of soda. And be sure to take 1 tablespoon of pure flax seed oil every morning with breakfast.

WEEK TWO | DAY 1

Breakfast

■ Cup **or** small bowl of broth only (no vegetables) from Dr. Rau's Alkaline Soup (page 152)

■ 4 ounces (½ cup) fresh grapefruit juice, preferably Ruby Red

■ 1 tablespoon pure flax seed oil

■ ¼ cup steel-cut oats cooked in 1 cup water with 1 date until very soft, about 15 minutes; no other sweetener

■ 1 small banana, sliced, **or** ½ cup Dried Fruit Compote (page 294)

■ 1 slice of spelt bread, toasted, with ½ teaspoon butter and 2 teaspoons your choice of naturally sweetened fruit preserves

■ 1 cup green tea **or** herb tea

Midmorning Snack

- ½ avocado with a squeeze of lemon juice

Lunch

- SALAD PLATE: Your choice of shredded raw vegetables dressed with lemon juice and extra virgin olive oil **or** ⅓ cup Shredded Beet and Carrot Salad (page 218); ⅓ cup shredded zucchini tossed with 1½ teaspoons fresh lemon juice and 1 teaspoon extra virgin olive oil; ½ cup Asian Sesame Slaw (page 219)

- 2 rye crisps

- STEAMED VEGETABLE PLATE: Broccoli florets, sliced carrots, and 1 small Yukon gold potato, sliced, all lightly steamed; do not over-cook. May splash with 2 teaspoons each lemon juice **or** balsamic vinegar and extra virgin olive oil **or** sunflower oil. Sprinkle with 1 tablespoon sunflower seeds.

Midafternoon Snack

- Small container (8 ounces) goat **or** sheep yogurt

Supper

- 4 ounces (½ cup) fresh carrot **or** other vegetable juice

- Cup of Dr. Rau's Alkaline Soup, including ⅓ cup diced vegetables from the soup

- ½ cup Olive Oil–Steamed Spinach (page 252)

- Twice-Baked Potatoes with Blue Cheese and Broccoli (page 252)

- Cup of herb tea, such as peppermint

Breakfast

- Same as Day 1, but instead of the butter and preserves with your toast, have ½ ounce of your favorite sheep cheese, such as Manchego, **or** goat cheese, such as Coach Farms brand; instead of the banana, have a small pear **or** peach

Midmorning Snack

- 1 small apple **or** a medium carrot

Lunch

- SALAD PLATE: Your choice of shredded raw vegetables dressed with lemon juice and extra virgin olive oil **or** 1 cup shredded romaine lettuce, 1 medium carrot, shredded, ¼ cup sliced cucumber, ¼ cup cooked chickpeas, tossed with 1 tablespoon each fresh lemon juice and extra virgin olive oil. Sprinkle 1 tablespoon feta cheese on top.

- STEAMED VEGETABLE PLATE: Cauliflower florets, green beans, and 1 small sweet potato, lightly steamed; do not overcook. May splash with 2 teaspoons each lemon juice **or** balsamic vinegar and extra virgin olive oil **or** sunflower oil. Sprinkle with 1 tablespoon pumpkin seeds.

- ½ cup Creamy Fruit Salad (page 292)

Midafternoon Snack

- With a cup of herb tea, enjoy 1 rye crisp with 1½ tablespoons Sweet Potato–Pine Nut Spread (page 186)

Supper

- 4 ounces (½ cup) fresh beet **or** other vegetable juice

- Bowl of Dr. Rau's Alkaline Soup, including ½ cup diced vegetables from the soup

- 1 cup steamed broccoli florets, dressed with fresh lemon juice and extra virgin olive oil

- ⅓ cup cooked basmati rice

- ⅓ cup Marinated Roasted Beets (page 219)

- Cup of herb tea

WEEK TWO | DAY 3

Breakfast

- Same as Day 1, but add 1 soft-boiled egg and eat your toast dry (you can dip it in the egg)

Midmorning Snack

- 5 cashews

Lunch

- SALAD PLATE: Your choice of shredded raw vegetables dressed with lemon juice and olive oil **or** ½ cup Swiss Potato Salad (page 224), made with no leek; ½ cup (loosely packed) alfalfa sprouts; ⅓ cup Shredded Beet and Carrot Salad

- STEAMED VEGETABLE PLATE: Swiss chard leaves, zucchini slices, and sliced peeled kohlrabi **or** celery root lightly steamed; do not over-cook. May splash with 2 teaspoons each lemon juice **or** balsamic vinegar and extra virgin olive oil **or** sunflower oil. Serve with 2 table-spoons cooked **or** sprouted lentils.

- 1 ripe pear, sliced, drizzled with 1½ teaspoons maple syrup and 1½ teaspoons chopped pecans

Midafternoon Snack

- 1 small cucumber, sliced, with 2 tablespoons Lemon-Rosemary White Bean Spread (page 192)

Supper

- 4 ounces (½ cup) fresh carrot **or** other vegetable juice

- Bowl Sweet Pea Soup with Fresh Mint (page 206), made with water **or** vegetable stock and no leek

- 1 slice of spelt bread

- 1 cup diced butternut squash and 1 cup loosely packed baby spinach leaves, steamed and tossed with balsamic vinegar and extra virgin olive oil

- Cup of herb tea

WEEK TWO | DAY 4

Breakfast

- Same as Day 1, but instead of a banana, have ½ mango, diced

Midmorning Snack

- 1 rye crisp spread with 2 teaspoons cashew butter and 1 teaspoon honey **or** 1 tablespoon Lemon-Rosemary White Bean Spread (page 192)

Lunch

- Either shredded vegetables of your choice tossed with lemon juice and extra virgin olive oil **or** ¼ recipe of Chopped Greek Salad (page 223)

- Bowl of Sweet Corn and Potato Chowder (page 202)

- ¾ cup mixed fruit salad of your choice **or** 1 apple

Midafternoon Snack

- 1 avocado sprinkled with lemon juice

Supper

- 4 ounces (½ cup) fresh beet **or** other vegetable juice

- Bowl of Dr. Rau's Alkaline Soup, including ½ cup diced vegetables from the soup

- Fennel Gratin (page 244)

- ⅓ cup cooked chestnuts

- ⅔ cup steamed Swiss chard leaves

- Cup of herb tea

WEEK TWO | DAY 5

Breakfast

- Same as Day 1

Midmorning Snack

- 1 carrot

Lunch

- SALAD PLATE: Your choice of shredded raw vegetables dressed with lemon juice and extra virgin olive oil **or** ½ cup raw **or** lightly steamed cauliflower florets, ¼ cup shredded carrot, and ¼ cup shredded zucchini **or** cucumber, and arugula leaves tossed with 2 teaspoons each lemon juice **or** balsamic vinegar and 2 teaspoons extra virgin olive oil **or** sunflower oil. Sprinkle 1 tablespoon crumbled Roquefort cheese on top.

- 2 rye crisps

- STEAMED VEGETABLE PLATE: Halved Brussels sprouts **or** shredded cabbage, ½ cup sliced garnet yam **or** sweet potato and Swiss chard leaves, lightly steamed; do not overcook.

Midafternoon Snack

- ¼ cup Guacamole (page 187) with 6 Baked Tortilla Chips (page 188)

Supper

- 4 ounces (½ cup) fresh carrot **or** other vegetable juice

- Bowl of Dr. Rau's Alkaline Soup, including ⅓ cup diced vegetables from the soup

- 1 Black Bean Burger with Cashews and Carrots (page 268)

- Olive Oil–Steamed Spinach (page 252), as much as you like

- Cup of peppermint tea

WEEK TWO | DAY 6

Breakfast

- Same as Day 1; but instead of the banana, have 1 apple

Midmorning Snack

- 1 plum **or** small pear, depending on the season

Lunch

- SALAD PLATE: Shredded vegetables of your choice dressed with fresh lemon juice and extra virgin olive oil **or** Crunchy Salad with Sunflower Seeds and Zesty Sprouts (page 217)

- Eggplant Steaks with Sun-Dried Tomatoes and Olives (page 243)

- ½ cup (cooked) spelt pasta, tossed with 1 teaspoon olive oil

- As much steamed broccoli as you like

Midafternoon Snack

- Small container (8 ounces) goat **or** sheep yogurt

Supper

- 4 ounces (½ cup) fresh carrot **or** other vegetable juice

- Ruby Beet Soup (page 196)

- Steamed vegetable plate of your choice

- Small spelt roll

- Cup of herb tea

WEEK TWO | DAY 7

Breakfast

- Same as Day 1. Instead of butter and preserves, have a small slice of sheep **or** goat cheese with your toast

Midmorning Snack

- 1 small apple

Lunch

- SALAD PLATE: Shredded vegetables of your choice tossed with fresh lemon juice and extra virgin olive oil **or** Avocado Salad with Strawberry Sauce (page 214)

- Asparagus Stir-Fry with Swiss Chard and Carrots (page 240) **or** steamed vegetable plate of your choice

- ½ cup steamed basmati rice

- 2 slices of ripe pineapple

Midafternoon Snack

- ½ avocado with a squeeze of lemon juice

Supper

- 4 ounces (½ cup) fresh beet **or** other vegetable juice
- Bowl of Dr. Rau's Alkaline Soup, including diced vegetables from the soup
- Pasta with Broccoli Rabe and Feta Cheese (page 230), made with spelt pasta; omit the hot pepper
- Cup of herb tea

WEEK THREE

By now you should be highly energized. Get out and walk as much as you can. It will stimulate weight loss and is excellent for your health in general. Continue to drink all the fluids you are supposed to. Also, continue to take your Alkala or bicarbonate of soda each morning. Keep in mind that no matter what the menu, you can eat as much as you want of any steamed green vegetable.

WEEK THREE | DAY 1

Breakfast

- Cup **or** small bowl of broth only (no vegetables) from Dr. Rau's Alkaline Soup (page 152)
- 4 ounces (½ cup) fresh grapefruit juice, preferably Ruby Red
- 1 tablespoon pure flax seed oil
- ⅓ cup steel-cut oats cooked in 1 cup water with 1 date until very soft, about 15 minutes; no other sweetener
- 1 small banana, sliced, **or** ½ cup Dried Fruit Compote (page 294)
- 1 slice of spelt bread, toasted, with ½ ounce goat **or** sheep cheese of your choice
- 1 cup of green tea **or** your favorite herb tea

Midmorning Snack

- 1 rye crisp with 2 teaspoons cashew butter and 1 teaspoon honey

Lunch

- SALAD PLATE: Your choice of shredded raw vegetables dressed with lemon juice and extra virgin olive oil **or** ⅓ cup Shredded Beet and Carrot Salad (page 218); ⅓ cup shredded zucchini tossed with 1½ teaspoons fresh lemon juice, 1 teaspoon extra virgin olive oil, and 2 teaspoons sunflower seeds; ½ cup Asian Sesame Slaw (page 219)

- Braised Kale with Carrots and Potatoes (page 245), made with vegetable stock

- Maple Baked Apple (page 289) **or** your choice of fresh fruit

Midafternoon Snack

- Cucumber and carrot sticks with ¼ cup Lemony Hummus with Toasted Cumin Seeds (page 188)

Supper

- 4 ounces (½ cup) fresh carrot **or** other vegetable juice

- Bowl of Dr. Rau's Alkaline Soup, including diced vegetables from the soup

- STEAMED VEGETABLE PLATE of your choice; as much greens as you like

- ½ cup cooked quinoa tossed with a drizzle of Asian sesame oil and a splash of wheat-free tamari

- Slice of spelt bread with 1 teaspoon butter **or** a drizzle of extra virgin olive oil

- Cup of herb tea

Breakfast

- Same as Day 1; include 1 soft-boiled egg; instead of the banana, have 1 apple

Midmorning Snack

- ½ avocado, with a squeeze of lemon juice

Lunch

- SALAD PLATE: Cucumbers stuffed with goat cheese, Swiss Potato Salad (page 224), and ½ cup mixed shredded carrot and zucchini tossed with freshly squeezed lemon juice and extra virgin olive oil

- STEAMED VEGETABLE PLATE of your choice

- Small spelt roll **or** slice of rye bread

- Frozen Banana-Maple Mousse (page 287)

Midafternoon Snack

- 1 carrot **or** 1 rye crisp with 2 tablespoons Sweet Potato–Pine Nut Spread (page 186)

Supper

- 4 ounces (½ cup) fresh beet **or** other vegetable juice

- Savory White Bean Soup (page 210)

- As much Olive Oil–Steamed Spinach (page 252) as you like

- Cup of herb tea

- 2 Maple-Pecan Cookies (page 286)

Breakfast

- ▣ Same as Day 1

Midmorning Snack

- ▣ 1 apple

Lunch

- ▣ SALAD PLATE: Mixed baby greens with thinly sliced cucumber, Marinated Roasted Beets (page 219), and shredded carrots with fresh dill

- ▣ Asparagus Risotto (page 237), served with 1 tablespoon grated Pecorino Romano cheese

Midafternoon Snack

- ▣ Small container (8 ounces) goat **or** sheep yogurt

Supper

- ▣ Small bowl of Lentil Soup (page 203)

- ▣ Baked sweet potato mashed with 2 teaspoons pumpkin seed oil **or** sunflower oil and 1 teaspoon maple syrup

- ▣ Steamed escarole with extra virgin olive oil and freshly squeezed lemon juice

- ▣ Cup of herb tea

Breakfast

- ▣ Same as Day 1. Substitute a peach **or** pear for the banana.

Midmorning Snack

- 1 carrot

Lunch

- Salad plate of your choice

- Succotash with Corn, Zucchini, and Green Beans (page 262)

- ½ cup steamed basmati rice

Midafternoon Snack

- ½ avocado with a squeeze of fresh lemon

Supper

- Bowl of Dr. Rau's Alkaline Soup, including ½ cup diced vegetables from the soup

- As much steamed broccoli as you like, dressed with extra virgin olive oil and fresh lemon juice

- Pita Pizzettes with Basil Goat Cheese and Black Olive Tapenade (page 190), made with spelt pita bread

- Cup of herb tea

WEEK THREE | DAY 5

Breakfast

- Same as Day 2

Midmorning Snack

- 5 cooked chestnuts

Lunch

- SALAD PLATE: Your choice of shredded raw vegetables tossed with freshly squeezed lemon juice and extra virgin olive oil **or** Celery Rémoulade (page 216)

- Sesame Quinoa with Bok Choy (page 242), made without the mushrooms

- Peachy Mango Mousse (page 287) **or** a piece of fresh fruit of your choice

Midafternoon Snack

- Cucumber slices, with ¼ cup Lemony Hummus

Supper

- 4 ounces (½ cup) fresh beet **or** other vegetable juice

- Bowl of Carrot-Ginger Soup (page 199)

- Steamed vegetable plate of your choice

- Spelt roll with 1 teaspoon butter and ½ ounce goat **or** sheep cheese

- Cup of herb tea

WEEK THREE | DAY 6

Breakfast

- Same as Day 1

Midmorning Snack

- 1 apple

Lunch

- SALAD PLATE: Your choice of shredded raw vegetables dressed with lemon juice and extra virgin olive oil **or** ½ cup Swiss Potato Salad (page 224), made with no leek; 1 cup (loosely packed) arugula dressed with balsamic vinegar and olive oil and ½ cup Shredded Beet and Carrot Salad (page 218)

- Creamy Polenta with Manchego Cheese (page 239)

- Steamed asparagus, drizzled with fresh lemon juice and extra virgin olive oil

Midafternoon Snack

- 5 cashews

Supper

- 4 ounces (½ cup) fresh carrot **or** other vegetable juice

- Lentils with Goat Cheese and Sun-Dried Tomatoes (page 246)

- Dried Fruit Compote (page 294)

- Cup of herb tea

WEEK THREE | DAY 7

Breakfast

- Same as Day 1; instead of the banana, have 1 peach **or** apple

Midmorning Snack

- 1 rye crisp with 2 tablespoons Sweet Potato–Pine Nut Spread (page 186)

Lunch

- Tossed green salad with shredded carrot, shredded zucchini, and cucumber slices

- Pecan-Crusted Catfish Fillets with Pineapple Slaw (page 278)

- Boiled new potatoes

- Steamed spinach

Midafternoon Snack

- 1 plum **or** carrot

Supper

- 4 ounces (½ cup) fresh beet **or** other vegetable juice

- Pasta Primavera (page 231)

- Steamed broccoli rabe, with a drizzle of extra virgin olive oil and fresh lemon juice

- Irene's Famous Lemon Tart (page 283)

- Cup of herb tea

Some Things You May Feel During and After the Swiss Detox Diet

Most people experience results very quickly. Many report a change in their digestion within a few days. On the second day, some but not all people feel a little malaise or even mild flulike symptoms. This is merely an indication that your body is beginning its internal transformation, and the first toxins have been dislodged and are circulating before being expelled. These symptoms will disappear within 24 hours.

More specifically, you may feel lighter, less bloated, or less stuffed after eating, and you may experience less flatulence. Because your body is detoxifying and you are eating more vegetables than you probably have before and drinking a lot of fluids, you will likely find you go to the bathroom very often; this is completely normal.

Hunger pangs between meals will disappear. That's because the plan avoids refined carbohydrates, which cause sudden swings in blood sugar, and feeds you lots of high-fiber vegetables like carrots and beets, which release their sugars slowly over the course of the day, keeping your blood sugar at an efficient, even level. The diet also includes two light, healthy snacks a day in between meals to make sure you remain on an even keel. If you suffer from acid indigestion or acid reflux, your symptoms will diminish. After five to seven days, you will feel calmer. Relieving food allergies is a great antidepressant.

In less than two weeks, many people notice a marked increase in their energy level. You'll sleep better—deeper and more relaxed—and wake up alert and refreshed, ready to go, with a spring in your step. A lot of this is because you will have eliminated many of the toxins that were slowly poisoning your system. Your body is also being fueled with all the good nutrients it needs.

By the end of the third week, when the immune system has had a chance to renew itself, the process really kicks in. You may notice you don't get sick as often. All those little colds and sniffles and minor flus going around don't stick. If you're suffering from a more serious chronic illness, there's a good chance your symptoms will lessen. And if you repeat this second stage for another three weeks, you will get much more marked results. Weight loss, if you need it, will be rapid. But more importantly, you'll notice a glow in your complexion and you'll feel as good as possible. The next chapter will explain one reason why.

You have done wonderful things for your body this week. By purging your system, shifting from an acid to an alkaline balance, and completely eliminating all the things that are bad for you, your body has been given a chance to rejuvenate itself. Going forward, we're going to continue the good work.

The challenge when you move to the permanent stage of my nutritional plan, the Maintenance Diet for Life, is to identify the food allergies that are unique to your body. You don't want to undo all the hard work you've begun. So before you begin the maintenance stage, let's examine what we mean by food allergies in this context.

CHAPTER SEVEN

Understanding Food Allergies

HIDDEN INTOLERANCES THAT MAY BE
AFFECTING YOUR HEALTH

When you initially begin Dr. Rau's Way with the Swiss Detox Diet, a number of foods are absolutely forbidden. These include all cow dairy products, including milk, yogurt, cheese, and ice cream; eggs; most grains containing gluten; white sugar and other refined carbohydrates; most nuts; and all seafood and meat, including chicken. The second and third weeks of the Swiss Detox Diet continue with a similar diet, adding in only certain wheat products and a little more protein. When you move on to the Maintenance Diet for Life, you may add a wider assortment of foods to your menus, but it's essential that you do so with great discrimination and care.

Although there are several reasons for avoiding some of the foods just noted, the prime purpose for not eating many of them is to eliminate 90 percent of known food allergens from your diet. These allergies are not the familiar histamine reactions that trigger nausea, an instant rash, or a choking sensation right after you eat something like shellfish or peanuts, or the kind of reaction many people get from bee stings. We call these triggers *secondary allergies*.

The allergies my diet targets are immunoglobulin-bound or T cell allergies of the slow type that arise from within your immune system. They take anywhere from one to three days to express themselves, and they are what we call *primary food allergies.*

The primary allergy results in a tremendous range of symptoms, which can vary from sluggishness to lack of focus and fatigue to indigestion, migraines, and sinus infections. Over time, these symptoms develop into full-blown chronic diseases.

These primary allergies are connected with specific proteins in the foods you eat, and most likely they were contracted during the first 18 months of your life. This may give you a clue to why so many people have a primary allergy to cow's milk and all the dairy products made from it.

Why No Cow Dairy

Of all the primary food allergies, cow dairy is the one that probably affects the largest number of people most acutely. That's because for a generation or two, especially in the United States and Canada, the vast majority of babies never saw their mother's breast. The baby boomer generation—that is, people born between 1946 and 1964—entered a brave new world of modern conveniences, including the baby bottle and artificial formula blended with cow's milk. I believe these "advancements" are in large part responsible for so many colicky babies and a generation beset with ear infections and tonsillitis. Let me explain.

Infants are born with relatively porous intestines, a natural version of what in adults we call "leaky gut syndrome," when damage to the good bacteria and mucous membranes of the intestines creates tiny lesions, or holes, allowing foreign matter to pass through. For the infant, this condition is not only normal but essential. The baby needs to easily absorb everything that comes in. After all, the infant is growing at an astounding pace, often doubling its weight in six months and tripling it within a year. Infants require all the nutrients they can get for such robust development.

Mother's milk offers the perfect nourishment for her infant. It passes easily through the intestinal walls and is absorbed seamlessly by the child. At the same time, besides nourishment, the baby is picking up valuable immunities from the mother. Breast-feeding a baby for 18 months to 2 years is a good way of ensuring the child's good health, especially for a strong immune system and prevention of allergies for life.

When breast-feeding is not chosen or is not possible as an option, most babies are given a formula based on cow's milk. The problem with this is that while, indeed, the milk passes right through the baby's gut and some of it is used as a nutrient, genetically, the human baby is pro-grammed to digest only human breast milk. While all the cow proteins pass through the baby's porous intestines, many of them, which are not found in human breast milk, are recognized as foreign substances by the part of the baby's immune system that resides along the lining of the small intestine, where nutrients are absorbed into the bloodstream.

This intestinal immune system is called the Peyer's patches—tiny lymph glands, which make up 80 percent of our entire immune system. In a baby, it makes up closer to 98 percent of the immune system; and when foreign proteins are detected, it produces powerful antigens against them.

Exposure after 18 months does not cause the same primary allergy because by then the gut has closed up, so instead of penetrating, these large foreign protein molecules are stopped and digested before absorp-tion. With this better-developed digestion, the foreign proteins are enzy-matically downgraded to their component amino acids, which are no longer allergenic.

These antigens created early in life from reaction to foreign proteins are essentially memory cells. They act as strict border guards. It's as if they had wanted posters tacked up on a bulletin board so they could instantly recognize alien invaders. You could think of them as security forces searching your bags, just like at the airport. They're looking for foods that are not allowed in—for which you have a genetic intolerance or that in the past have caused you difficulty. These border guards are charged with screening out troublesome substances before they enter your system.

THE PROBLEM WITH COW'S MILK

The following table compares cow's milk and human breast milk. Notice that in addition to containing *more* protein, the cow's milk is made up of a large amount of *wrong* protein. Compared with human milk, it also has way too much phosphorous, which binds with the calcium, making it impossible to utilize the calcium properly. And we know that phosphorous in this excessive amount is irritating to the brain and nervous system. That's why babies given cow's milk often cry not long after feeding.

MILK (Per 100 grams whole milk)

COMPONENT	COW	HUMAN MOTHER
Protein:	3.5 g	1.1 g
Fat:	3.5 g	4.0 g
Carbohydrate:	4.9 g	9.5 g
Calcium:	118 mg	33 mg
Phosphorous:	93 mg	4 mg
Vitamin C:	1 mg	5 mg

Through her breast milk, the mother also offers the baby her individualized immune protection. When I was a little boy, our neighbor kept a few cows. In the evenings, I would go into the barn with a pail and visit and get milk from my favorite cow. This cow was living in the same surroundings we did; she ate pure grass in summer and locally cut hay in the winter, both of which had no chemicals or fertilizers. Today, commercial cow's milk is blended at the factory from many animals from different herds. Consequently, the baby who drinks this milk is receiving immunological information from an average of 30,000 animals, which today are housed in a totally unnatural life situation. Unless from an isolated organic herd, cow's milk confers immunological confusion as well. Imagine a baby's immature, not-yet-developed immune system being confronted with the DNA from thousands of cows!

Each and every time the Peyer's patches see one of these alien proteins, they get up in arms, which results in a highly inflamed intestinal mucosa and damage to the good bacteria that both promote digestion and protect the gut. Because the primary allergen is ingested day after day, eventually the gut and the flora that line it are so damaged that tiny lesions occur in the delicate, thin wall of the intestine. This is the condition we refer to as "leaky gut syndrome," and it can wreak havoc with your intestinal immune system.

Secondary allergies develop because the damaged intestinal membranes are so leaky that other large molecules, not yet fully digested, are able to pass through, where they get recognized as foreign. So these secondary allergies can develop at any time in your life and are noticed because they are normally histamine bound. That means they are triggered not by the Peyer's patches, but by mast cells (found mostly in connective tissues) which release histamines. The reaction is often quick and somewhat dramatic: nausea, a rash, swelling particularly of the throat, severe headache. Most people are aware of their secondary allergies.

The primary food allergies, on the other hand, are a bit insidious and hard to identify, because unlike secondary histamine allergies, which hit us at once, these take one to three days to express themselves. That's why you typically don't connect the symptom with the food you are allergic to. If it's a common food that you eat almost every day, the symptoms will always be present, gradually building up over time.

You can repair the damage to and atrophy of your gut if you avoid the primary food allergy for a considerable length of time—three weeks being the bare minimum. After several weeks or sometimes a couple of months, the intestinal membranes regenerate so that they have more density, more surface, and more useful, protective intestinal bacteria. Therefore, after a minimum of three, and preferably six weeks, of complete avoidance of primary food allergies, the intestinal membrane has been rebuilt and shows more tolerance to your allergen. However, keep in mind that this primary allergy remains with you always; and the allergen must be avoided for life.

A wonderful benefit of my nutritional plan is that if you follow it

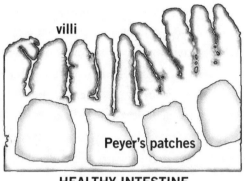

HEALTHY INTESTINE

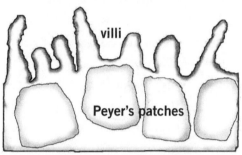

DISEASED INTESTINE

over time and heal your intestinal mucosa by avoiding primary allergies and by up-building the intestinal bacteria, which protect the delicate walls of the gut, your secondary allergies will disappear.

Food Allergies Disarm Your Natural Defenses

If you've mobilized 80 percent of your immunological army to defend against damaging food allergies, there will not be enough troops available to fight all the other important immunological battles—against infections and even cancer. In addition, due to the inflammatory damage from primary allergies, the surface area of the intestines, vital for absorbing the good nutrients you need, is reduced.

Another scenario is that an overactive immune system can spin out of control. After years of entanglement with the primary allergies, the remaining troops will be so sensitive to any invasion—trigger-happy, if you will—that at the slightest provocation they start to attack their own organs, which leads to all the autoimmune diseases like allergies, lupus, multiple sclerosis, arthritis, and chronic skin conditions such as eczema and psoriasis. While symptoms may come on us suddenly, appearing seemingly out of nowhere, in fact there is a good chance they have been building up for years.

This explains again why nutrition is such an important part of my healing for a wide range of symptoms and diseases. Without calming down the intestinal immune system, you'll never be successful at treating major chronic and degenerative diseases.

There are a number of misconceptions involving allergies. One is that you can build up tolerance. To the contrary, there is a threshold to any allergy that becomes *lower* with each exposure. Except in cases of certain genetic diseases, your immune system usually handles a first mild encounter with little effort. But each time your defenses confront the same offending allergen, their state of alert gets higher and higher because the recognition is much keener. They've already got the wanted poster on the wall and so can react much faster.

When your immune system is exposed to the same foods you are allergic to over and over again, often for many years, the physical consequences become worse and worse, like a giant wave gathering height as it nears the shore. Once you have been flooded, as it were, and symptoms take hold, it requires a minimum of three weeks just to begin the cleanup. Then you have to rebuild. Completely desensitizing an irritated immune system can take months or even years. If you want to stay healthy and ward off systemic diseases, there are many foods you may need to avoid for a lifetime. But that is a benefit, not a liability.

So many people with allergies never recover; they simply visit their doctor for shots to quell superficial symptoms every week or every month. Over time, the assault of the allergens on the immune system still

DR. RAU'S WAY CONQUERS FOOD ALLERGIES

Like subclinical infections, primary T cell food allergies we are not even aware of are largely responsible for a tremendous number of specific illnesses and many of the problematic symptoms almost every person experiences: headaches, stomachaches, bloating, depression, sinus problems, inability to focus, insomnia, or that uncomfortable feeling of just being "out of sorts."

- **The Swiss Detox Diet** allows a rich vegetarian diet but eliminates about 90 percent of known food allergens. Many people are surprised when they discover their food allergies or intolerances because most of these substances have been doing their damage silently for many years.

- **My Maintenance Diet for Life,** the stage at which you are allowed greater choices and assume responsibility for choosing the right foods, still avoids around 80 percent of primary food allergens.

What is so interesting is that once you have gone through the detoxifying program and have given your intestinal mucous membranes a chance to heal, secondary histamine allergies are no longer of as much importance.

takes its toll. The marvelous thing about Swiss biological medicine is that it takes aim at the root cause of the allergic reactions. You bring about the cure yourself through the choices you make of what to eat.

Of course, the only way to do this is first to recognize what you are allergic to and then avoid those foods diligently. At Paracelsus Clinic Lustmühle, we have special blood tests that can identify each individual's allergen profile. It is a quick, efficient way to learn at a glance what your system can and cannot tolerate.

But if you cannot find your way to a clinic, my Swiss Detox Diet will give your immune system a clean slate, especially if you choose to remain on the program for six or even nine weeks. With this clean slate, you can more easily recognize when your body is adversely reacting to a particular food. But you must become attuned to your body and pay attention to how it responds when you introduce new things to your diet. Unlike the sudden violent symptoms of histamine reactions, T cell immune system allergies can be subtle at first, and they often take three or even four days to manifest themselves. Most people are not even aware they have these food allergies, because they don't make the connection.

Not only is there a time lag before symptoms appear, but the effects differ greatly from person to person. Allergic reactions may range anywhere from headache, diarrhea, and aching in the joints to fatigue, inability to focus, and insomnia. Because of our individual genetic compositions, we all have certain physical weaknesses. That is usually where an allergy will strike first.

Food allergies that overstimulate the immune system almost always have serious consequences of one sort or another, because they build up over time. Day by day, starting when you are very young, the allergy gets worse and worse, because you don't even know you have a problem and you keep eating the same food. It's not that the symptoms aren't there; it's that you don't connect them to the food you eat.

Eventually, the entire immune system weakens, which results in a range of serious symptoms. As explained earlier, an immune system allergy expresses itself either as an irritation of the mucous membranes—in which case it will manifest itself with problems like a sinus infection, a migraine headache, allergies, bronchitis, asthma, or chronic pneumonia—or it will affect the entire immune system, which can lead to chronic fatigue syndrome, thyroid deficiencies, chronic skin conditions like eczema, and even cancer.

Another fallacy about foods and allergies is the deep-seated belief that our body will tell us what it needs. It's a fairy tale that we should eat what we crave. Ironically, we tend to crave the very foods we are most allergic to. You're getting all the calories, protein, and other nutrients you need, so why this urge? Because these allergens irritate the intestinal mucosae, which can stimulate the production of serotonin, an enzyme that is produced in the gut, but that acts on the brain. And serotonin gives us a feeling of well-being or pleasure.

Intolerance for a certain food (or foods) may be genetic—that is, built into our genes. Or as is common, it may be that you were given too much of a particular food when you were too young, before your gastrointestinal system was equipped to process it. Consequently, powerful antibodies developed against it. That's why it's important to breast-feed babies and not give them solid food before they are physically ready for it.

No matter how your intolerances became allergies in the first place, it's best to avoid them as much as possible. They can only get worse. So how do you go about recognizing what you shouldn't eat?

Once you have detoxified and cleaned out the allergens from your gastrointestinal system, you'll want to add back foods slowly, one at a time, paying close attention over the following three or four days. I suggest you begin with wheat, because that is such an important part of our Western diet and is prevalent in so many forms, including bread, crackers, pasta, cereal, and flour.

Celiac disease is an extremely serious genetic intolerance to gluten, a protein found in many grains, though especially in wheat. If you are an adult and you have it, you know it. It would have been diagnosed when you were a young child. The wheat allergy we are looking for is one of the immune system. To see if it is there or not, during the Swiss Detox Diet we clean out our system by eating bread and crackers made with spelt flour.

Spelt is an ancestor of our modern wheat. It is a grain that has undergone less genetic engineering, causes far fewer allergic reactions, and contains enzymes that actually boost the immune system. During the Swiss Detox Diet, you can also enjoy cornmeal, buckwheat, amaranth, and quinoa, all of which are gluten free.

After you have completely detoxified and are ready to proceed to the Maintenance Diet for Life, go back to the three-week program and choose any meal you like. Or you can mix and match the selections. But in addition, have a slice of whole wheat or whole-grain bread; white bread is never on my diet. The next day and the day after that, continue with the Swiss Detox Diet, eating only pure, simply prepared foods. Pay close attention to how you feel.

Think like a hypochondriac during these few days. If you notice anything—from a sinus headache or indigestion to depression or even a vague malaise—have another piece of bread, or two, and see what happens in another few days. If after that time you notice nothing out of the usual, go on to the next food you want to try.

In general, we find people who are intolerant to domestic American wheat sometimes do better with imported pure semolina pasta. High-quality ingredients are usually tolerated better because they contain a smaller gene pool. There is less for your immune receptors to deal with. If you eat a fine cheese produced by a serious cheese-maker, you are likely confronting the gene pool of a single herd. If you eat a mass-produced cheese, you may be dealing with different DNA from thousands of animals whose milk is collected from hundreds of different dairies.

In addition, when you choose artisanally produced foods of the highest

TIPS FOR AVOIDING DIETARY ALLERGIC REACTIONS

- Rotate what you eat. There is safety in numbers. Aside from providing all the nutrients you need, a variety of foods protects against repeated contact with any food allergy.

- Do not eat the same foods all the time. If you develop a compulsive craving, consider it a warning sign.

- Avoid processed foods, genetically engineered crops, and artificial ingredients, which can trigger severe allergic reactions.

- Pay attention to unexplained malaise and other undiagnosed symptoms. Try to see if there is any correlation between how you feel and what you eat.

quality, you lessen the chance of encountering a genetically modified product, which I urge you to avoid. Incomplete testing has been done on these Frankenstein crops, and we have no idea of their long-term consequences in the human body.

Other foods that tend to cause problems are different kinds of mushrooms, nuts, and dairy products. Milk is for baby animals and is not a beverage adults should drink; it is far too dense in proteins. So when I say *dairy*, I am referring to cheese, butter, yogurt, and cream. I don't recommend milk at all.

Most people digest goat dairy easily. The same is true of sheep milk. Some people tolerate water buffalo milk well, which does make a fine mozzarella; others have a hard time digesting it. Often people who are allergic to cow dairy also react to water buffalo. You must feel your way ingredient by ingredient and act like your very own detective investigating yourself.

When it comes to food allergies, however, there is one class of foods that can be considered guilty until proven innocent: cow dairy products. Given that cow's milk was given to many American babies, particularly of the "boomer" generation, in bottles since birth, poured into bowls of cereal each day, and foisted on them in tall glasses at every meal—with the misguided promise of strong bones—it's no wonder this is one of the leading food allergies of our day. If you are allergic to cow's milk, most likely it is an intolerance that has been growing worse and worse your entire life. Every time you drink a glass of cow's milk, eat a container of yogurt or cottage cheese, or dig into a slab of Cheddar, your immune system is assaulted. Most people who believe they are lactose intolerant are actually suffering from an allergy to the proteins in the milk, not the lactose, which is a simple sugar.

Women in particular are beset with this problem because before and during menopause, to avoid osteoporosis they are strongly encouraged by their doctors—and the dairy industry, which has a very powerful lobby—to drink excessive amounts of milk. And look at all the symptoms that crop up at this time in their life: fatigue, depression, lack of muscle strength, indigestion, acid reflux, insomnia, thyroid insufficiency.

Most doctors—and their unsuspecting patients—chalk up these ailments to that "time of life" and loss of hormones. The reality is that most of their problems probably stem from the milk. It's both the cause of a strong T cell allergic reaction and is adding to protein overload, leading to acidity in the blood. That is what is preventing these women from leading a vital, energetic life.

Understanding Osteoporosis

Whenever you say no milk, people worry about where to get their calcium. Avoiding bone loss that leads to osteoporosis is a very serious matter. Some bone degeneration inevitably occurs with age, especially in women, but osteoporosis is a debilitating condition that can usually be avoided. It results when so much calcium and minerals are lost from the bone that the structural integrity of the bone itself is compromised. That's what's meant by *low bone density*. This fragility often leads to stress fractures of the hip, spine, and wrist. Besides being exceedingly painful, it is actually a life-threatening illness. But neither milk nor calcium supplements are the answer.

Not long ago, the Women's Health Initiative, one of the largest and longest epidemiological medical studies ever undertaken in the United States, shocked the public by announcing that taking calcium supplements had no effect on the rate of fractures in postmenopausal women. In fact, the rate of fractures was slightly higher than in the control group. Other studies showed the same to be true for women who drank copious amounts of milk. From a biological medicine point of view, this makes perfect sense.

Problems such as osteoporosis arise not from drinking too little milk, but from ingesting too much animal protein. As we learned in Chapter 5, it is acidity in the bloodstream caused by eating too much protein that leaches calcium and other minerals from the bones and cartilage. Numerous studies as far back as 1988 have documented this; though it is only recently, with the latest results, that the public is being made aware. Eating plenty of leafy green vegetables and whole grains will give you all the calcium you need. Combining this good diet with moderate weight-bearing exercise will result in healthy bones.

Now that you know what to look for with food allergies, you're ready to move on to my Maintenance Diet for Life, because good nutrition to support biological medicine is not a quick fix. If you're serious about healing and leading a vital life, don't stop just when you've begun to see results. Balancing your system and constantly lightening your toxic load is an intelligent and powerful way to lead a healthy and active life as long as you can.

CHAPTER EIGHT

Maintenance Diet for Life

THE BALANCING ACT CONTINUES

Maintenance is a very bland word for what is a very pleasing diet. What it means is that you are maintaining the internal balance you worked so hard to achieve with the Swiss Detox Diet: your internal alkaline balance, reduction of toxins, and lifting of the weight from your immune system. At the same time, since you will continue the diet for months—or years, we hope, for the good of your health and vitality—it is a diet filled with a variety of foods, so it's easy to maintain.

Many new tastes and textures are included. Much stays the same. Fresh vegetables and whole grains still make up the bedrock of your diet. Once you've learned just how delicious fresh organic vegetables can be, you probably won't want to give them up, anyway. But nonvegetarians who have followed Dr. Rau's Way to improve their health will welcome the additions to their meals. You can have more cheeses, yogurt, a few mushrooms, a greater variety of nuts, seasonings and spices, pasta, risotto, and a little—but not a lot—more sweets.

At this point, you can enjoy chicken and fish several times a week. A very small portion of lean organic beef or lamb once or twice a month will not harm you. Best of all, you can indulge, if you wish, with a cup of coffee each morning and an occasional glass of red wine with dinner in the evening. The diet remains easy in that there's still no counting of numbers and no calculations of amounts.

What's key to this stage of the diet is how you ease into it. As the discussion of food allergies in the previous chapter made clear, you must enlarge your palette of ingredients slowly so that you do not undo all the good of your recent detox. Identifying which foods agree with you and which cause problems will take some time. Of course, the state of your health has a lot to do with just how careful you need to be and how quickly the diet can progress.

As we've learned, this excellent nutrition is both preventative medicine and a powerful tool against all kinds of chronic inflammatory and degenerative diseases, including heart disease and cancer. It's also a potent buffer against the environment's toxic loads, such as mercury, air pollution, geophysical disturbances, and the stresses we deal with every day. So it is certainly worth making every effort. Knowing you can do so much to help yourself should be a great motivator. This chapter and the recipes later in the book are meant to be a guide. It's your job to find your own comfort level and to make Dr. Rau's Way work best for you.

Avoid all processed foods. They are filled with poisons, damaging trans fats, and preservatives. Once you become accustomed to pure natural ingredients, there's no going back. Your taste will become more acute and your palate more sophisticated. Seek out local organic farmers and suppliers of top-quality poultry, fish, and cheese. Eat produce in season, when it will be freshest and naturally taste best. Treat these ingredients simply and with respect. Being in tune with the earth around you is a good way to plan your meals. When you think about it, that's what the contemporary fine food movement is all about.

Certified organic fruits and vegetables are now raised under strict guidelines that prohibit chemicals and pesticides. They are invariably fresher and consequently more nutritious. That's because they are not bred solely for shelf life and sturdiness for shipping but for taste, and they often come from local growers. The difference between organic and tired commercial produce is not subtle.

HOW TO EAT FOR LIFE

You must have:
    A substantial breakfast

    A big lunch, with a nice raw salad as your first course. Whenever possible, lunch should be your largest meal of the day.

    A relatively light supper

In addition:
    You may have both a midmorning and midafternoon snack, if you need them. Raw fruit should not be eaten after 4:00 in the afternoon.

    Water and other beverages should be consumed between meals, not with your food. As on detox, you should continue to drink 2 to 3 liters of fluids a day.

    You may have a *small* glass of freshly squeezed juice in the morning, but fruit juice should not be drunk as a beverage. Orange juice in particular is full of sugar and highly acidic. Grapefruit juice should remain your first choice.

    A glass of wine is permitted with meals several times a week.

    You may have 1 cup of coffee or caffeinated tea in the morning. After that it's decaf or, preferably, herb teas. An exception is made for green tea. While caffeinated, it is an excellent antioxidant, but do not drink caffeinated green tea after 3:00 P.M., or you may have trouble sleeping.

Artisanally produced raw-milk goat and sheep cheeses are more healthful and tend to be produced under much more immaculate conditions than commercial pasteurized cheeses. Blue cheeses in particular, like Roquefort, with their natural penicillin, are good for you and support the intestinal flora.

Ideally, it would be best to have fish once or twice a week, especially oily fish, which is very rich in omega-3 essential oils. High-quality fresh fish is hard to come by in many places, though. Because of pollution, many species are contaminated with mercury and PCBs, and these are serious contaminants that are extremely difficult to remove from the body. Supermarkets with good seafood departments are responding with wild and organically farmed fish, and this is what you should look for. As a rule, Pacific fish are safer than fish from the Atlantic, and fish caught in cold, deep waters are more healthful. Avoid scavenger bottom feeders like monkfish and fish at the top of the food chain, like tuna and swordfish. Canned Nordic brisling sardines, which are rich in omega-3s, can supplement your diet in small amounts.

From a culinary point of view, meal planning is easy. Refer to pages 51–54 for a listing of what you must eat every day, what you can only eat once in a while, and what you should never eat. Using the Swiss Detox Diet as an outline, develop your own menus to enlarge the picture. You can enjoy recipes you've loved for years, as long as they don't contain any forbidden foods; or pick from the more than 100 easy and enticing recipes in this book. They are all Dr. Rau approved. My wife, Elisabeth, who is a nurse and who is extremely familiar with the nutritional program at the Paracelsus Clinic, personally reviewed each and every one.

The basis of my Maintenance Diet for Life includes a wide variety of fresh organic vegetables, fruits, and whole grains. You must continue to eat a substantial amount of raw and lightly steamed vegetables; by now you may have worked your way up to 50 percent raw. Now that you are on maintenance, you can even have a small salad at supper in addition to your other food, if you digest it well. You should also enjoy a range of whole grains, especially quinoa. These foods are rich in antioxidants, essential amino acids, and valuable omega-3 fatty acids, which are integral to cell integrity, nerve impulses, and metabolism.

Aside from all the vitamins, minerals, and trace elements you'll glean from these foods, the high fiber they contain ensures your good intestinal bacteria stay in peak form and that you receive maximum nutritional benefit from what you eat. Cow dairy products are expressly forbidden, although small amounts of butter and cream are permitted because they are mostly pure fat; they contain little protein. You may, however, enjoy moderate amounts of sheep and goat cheese and yogurt. It's a good idea to have two soft-boiled eggs a week to make sure you get enough lecithin.

Keep a variety of nuts and seeds handy for sprinkling on top of salads. Have a bowl of vegetable soup or chowder or a veggie burger. Accompany your meal with chewy whole-grain bread and a good sheep or goat cheese. Several times a week, you can enjoy a chicken dish or simply grilled or poached fish. Just be sure to keep portions small. Steamed vegetables are always a good choice; for the most part, you can eat as much of these as you like.

If you have no interest in cooking or are unwell and wish to eat as simply as possible, you can do that, too—even when you're eating out. Just opt for any salad or selection of shredded raw vegetables you're in the mood for, dressed with fresh lemon juice or mild vinegar and extra virgin olive or sunflower oil. Order lots of side vegetables.

Once you've spent a couple of months on my Maintenance Diet for Life, eating to support your health will be second nature. You'll be enjoying the way you eat as well as the way you feel so much that you'll wonder why it took so long to find a better way. You'll find that as you continue eating this way, your preferences will naturally shift toward what is good for you. The invigorating high energy level you will enjoy all day, maintained by so many good fresh fruits, vegetables, and whole grains, is a powerful motivator. Those sudden highs and depressing lows brought on by a sugar rush no longer have the same appeal. Still, who could live with themselves if they thought they would never taste chocolate ever again?

It's Impossible to Cheat

Some diets have ironclad rules that can't be broken. That's one reason why most people don't stay on them for very long. With Dr. Rau's

Way, it's impossible to cheat. If you have detoxified and followed the maintenance diet for several months, eating something forbidden will not hurt you.

We all have our guilty pleasures. And my patients know that when I say "none," I mean "very little." When I say "never," I mean "once in a very great while." This means that if you remain on the basic maintenance diet for months, or hopefully years, if you have a steak or a rack of lamb or a small slice of chocolate cake once in a great while, it shouldn't have a noticeable effect on your health.

When you celebrate a special occasion at a restaurant, are invited over to a friend's house for dinner, or wish to throw an elaborate party, you can eat almost anything for a night. Of course, the more fragile your health, the more careful you should be, because every little bit helps. But pleasure is a powerful force, and everyone needs a treat from time to time. Just don't make it a habit. Remember, we built a strong foundation for our nice brick house, and we don't want anything to knock it down.

If, on the other hand, you are away on a business trip or a long vacation and you eat everything you're not supposed to for too long, it's not good. But the damage can easily be repaired. Simply return to the Swiss Detox Diet for a week or two, and you will be back where you started. Never give up!

As a matter of fact, any time you feel you need a boost, because you've been ill, you feel your immune system needs a boost, or because you want to lose some weight, you can simply jump-start your system back to go even faster with my One-Week Intensive Cure (Chapter 10).

Breakfast, Lunch, and Dinner

You'll find my Maintenance Diet for Life is similar to the three-week detox program, though much more inclusive. But let's review the program again. First of all, forget about how you've structured your meals in the past. You're going to wake up and have a nice big, satisfying breakfast. Don't like to eat in the morning . . . just a cup of coffee and maybe a small glass of orange juice? That's just not an optimal way to eat.

Breakfast

Breakfast is the one of most important meals of the day, and it should be substantial. A Dr. Rau breakfast consists of a small (4-ounce) glass of freshly squeezed juice, preferably pink grapefruit, with pulp; a bowl of whole-grain cereal, cold or cooked, such as steel-cut oats or muesli; stewed and/or fresh fruit; and whole-grain bread with sheep or goat cheese or pure sugar-free fruit preserves, made with honey or natural fruit sweetener (not artificial sweeteners), if you like. Once or twice a week, you may add a soft-boiled egg or a small serving of goat or sheep yogurt.

Eating a healthy, substantial breakfast will make a big difference in your energy level, your ability to concentrate, your calmness and evenness of mood, your ability to fall asleep easily at night and sleep soundly, and the regularity of your digestive and elimination systems.

You probably won't be hungry for hours, but still the diet allows you a midmorning snack, if you're hungry. It could be something as simple as an apple or a couple of carrots, or it might be half an avocado spritzed with freshly squeezed lemon juice or a rye crisp or slice of toasted whole-grain bread with a tasty bean or sweet potato spread or a nut butter. This snack is often a good idea, because if you wait until you're starving at lunch, you'll be much more tempted to stuff anything in your mouth and not take the time to prepare or order a proper meal.

Lunch

Lunch, whenever possible, should be your most substantial meal. It's better to take in most of your protein requirements earlier in the day. Begin always with a salad of mostly raw vegetables; shredded root vegetables like carrots and beets and light alkaline vegetables like zucchini are particularly good choices. It will fill you up with a minimum of calories while providing valuable fiber, vitamins, minerals, proteins, and essential fatty acids. I encourage you to explore a more European kind of vegetarian *hors d'oeuvres variés*, as the French call it, with an enticing assortment of plain, dressed, and marinated vegetables, not just lettuce as in an American salad. The section called "The Salad Bar" (page 212) will teach you how to plan and execute this delicious part of the meal with a minimum of time and effort. Be sure to include a sprinkling of seeds, nuts, and sprouts, too.

The dressing of your salad is particularly important. Simply toss away all those bottles of processed dressings filled with preservatives, sugar, and other things you don't need. Extra virgin olive oil and fresh lemon juice, balsamic vinegar, or another mild vinegar should be what you drizzle on any kind of salad.

Then you get to enjoy a hot entree of your choice: a pasta, rice dish, veggie burger with sides, whatever you feel like. A selection of tempting main dishes are given later (page 227). You can even have dessert, if you want it. Just be sure it meets the principles of Dr. Rau's Way.

Dinner

Dinner should be relatively light: a soup, perhaps, with some bread and cheese or a light pasta dish. You can have a small salad, but opt in general for cooked, rather than raw foods in the evening, so your digestion is not stressed. If for logistic or social purposes a big meal just does not work at lunch, and dinner needs to be more substantial, at least try not to eat too late at night, and do not overeat.

What You May Feel

Your first month or two on the diet will probably surprise you. Even with the cleansing of the Swiss Detox Diet behind you, your body will still be making serious adjustments, and your immune system will continually be strengthening. Changes in your metabolism, your digestion, and your energy level will be noticeable. You'll feel as if you are eating more food than ever before; but if you need to, you will still lose weight.

So many vegetables and whole grains may cause some changes in your digestion. You may find you develop mild diarrhea or defecate frequently even once you reach maintenance. This is perfectly normal and to be expected. After all, you are completely remaking the internal landscape of your intestines, and you are still purging toxins. Where do you think those poisons go? Most are filtered through the liver and eliminated through the bowel.

If your symptoms are severe, cut back on the raw fruits and vegetables a little, but not too much. They are essential for the efficacy of the program. Don't worry if you defecate more often than usual for up to two months. The truth is, once you are regulated internally, you will be as regular as clockwork—a blessing for many patients who struggled with constipation and irregularity for years. Continue to increase the raw vegetables gradually until you are at as close to a 50:50 balance of raw and cooked food as is comfortable for you, and you feel in peak form. I guarantee, once your internal environment is balanced, you will feel—and look—better than you ever imagined.

What's Off-Limits?

In some ways, changing the way you eat, trying it Dr. Rau's Way, is much easier than you'd think. But you are going to have to learn to live without some formerly favorite foods. What are you giving up? Read on.

Refined Sugar

White sugar causes the glucose in your bloodstream to skyrocket and then crash. In addition, white sugar is refined through a process that uses arsenic, and even tiny trace amounts add to your toxic load.

White Flour

Refined flour is completely devoid of the nutritional content of the inner germ and the fiber of the outer husk of the grain. It is a food basically devoid of redeeming characteristics. Once you've moved on to maintenance, whole wheat or other whole-grain breads are fine if you tolerate them well.

Cow Dairy Products

The only cow dairy allowed are small amounts of organic butter and cream from time to time, because my concern is with the proteins, not the fat. Even if you are not allergic to cow's milk, I discourage its use. Because of the way milk is collected, processed, and distributed in the United States, it is a possible source of many contaminants, not least being the artificial estrogen DES given to cows to boost their milk production on large corporate farms. This drug causes unexplained infertility in humans as well as cancer, and traces are present in the milk of cows treated. To allay any concerns you have about calcium, read all about osteoporosis on page 116.

I recommend, instead, sheep and goat cheeses. Excellent mild yogurts with active cultures are made from both these types of milk as well as a wide range of cheeses to suit all purposes.

Meat

Without even dealing with the humanitarian aspects, the flesh of any four-legged animal is best not eaten. Meat is dense in proteins and thus highly acidic. Despite the fact it is a so-called complete protein, it is proportionately low in the important essential amino acids, so the quality is not what we are looking for. Red meats also contain a lot of saturated fat that contributes to high cholesterol. And there is ample evidence that bovine spongiform encephalopathy (BSE), popularly called mad cow disease, is much more prevalent than the meat industry would like us to think. The U.S. government seems to have a don't ask, don't tell policy toward beef cattle: Don't inspect and don't know. That's quite a gamble.

If upon rare occasion you do eat a small serving of beef or lamb, make sure it is from an organically raised animal fed nothing but vegetable feed with no antibiotics and no hormones. If you have a choice, opt for one of the leaner cuts, such as fillet of beef or tenderloin of lamb, and be sure you eat only a little bit—a 3- or 4-ounce portion, not a 6- or 8-ounce slab of meat.

Pork, including bacon and sausages, is off limits completely. I know this is a hard one for many people, but the reasons are multifold. Some pork products are too high in saturated fat; some are too lean and hence have a high amino acid content. Also, pork is high in histamines, which aggravate the immune system, and in sulfur, an element that attracts free radicals that can form carcinogens within the body.

If you must have sausage, reach for a high-quality chicken sausage instead, but be sure you read the label. Again, you're looking for a pure product: no sugar, preservatives, or artificial chemicals.

Also avoid game, including venison and rabbit. All these wild meats are high in histamines, and they contain too much protein.

Seafood

Shrimp, lobster, crab, oysters, mussels, and clams all present hidden forms of dangerous toxins, such as PCBs, and heavy-metal contamination. Remember, these creatures live at the bottom of the ocean, where all sediment falls, and they filter the seawater through their bodies. All shellfish should be strenuously avoided.

The same goes for large ocean fish, such as tuna and swordfish, and bottom feeders like monkfish, especially from the Atlantic, which is sadly polluted. Beware, too, of so-called farmed fish, especially salmon, which have been measured to contain high amounts of PCBs. Wild

Pacific or freshwater fish from sustainable farmed or clean locations are your safest choices. In America, environmental groups like Oceans Alive periodically issue updated lists about which fish are safe and ethical to eat.

Processed Foods

Quite simply, these are poisons. The same chemicals that keep packaged foods from spoiling for months, if not years, will remain inert in your body, resisting elimination, forming free radicals, and greatly increasing your toxic load. Many additives are carcinogenic. Learning to eat fresh, natural foods is one of the basic tenets of Dr. Rau's Way.

Onions

As hard as this may seem, onions are an irritant to many people and can cause thickening of the lymph fluids. Instead, use small amounts of leek, garlic, and chives.

Table Salt

Ordinary table salt, as mentioned before, contains preservatives and additives that are not good for you. Sea salt and Himalayan salt are fine, used in moderation.

In some ways, changing the way you eat, trying it Dr. Rau's Way, is much easier than you'd think. At first, any change feels challenging; studies have shown that even good change is stressful. But once you get used to it, you will be surprised at how much you enjoy your new, healthful way of eating. Because not only will you feel better than you ever have before, you may well find a new appreciation for the pure, natural flavors of foods. If cooking and dining out are important parts of your life, you won't have to sacrifice much. In fact, you may find eating even more pleasurable once it becomes a regular part of your healing program.

Eating Out When You're on Maintenance

Following the diet at home really becomes simple once you've adjusted your pantry and your menus. If you have lunch at your desk, it's fairly easy to bring your home food to the office. Salads with dressing on the side transport easily in covered containers. Containers of goat or sheep yogurt take the place of cow. Steamed vegetables and many vegetarian main courses are quite portable and less subject to spoilage than meat-based dishes. They are usually good either warm or at room temperature. You can keep small bottles of extra virgin olive oil and balsamic vinegar in your desk, and lemons are easy to carry. Eating out is a bit more challenging.

Take a look at any restaurant menu these days, though, and you will see plenty of vegetarian options. Almost all fine restaurants offer at least a couple of vegetarian main courses, not to speak of soups, salads, and pastas. In a pinch, you can create your own vegetable plate by ordering several sides. Just ask the waiter to plate them together.

And then there's the fact that you are allowed fish and chicken several times a week. The only problem with restaurants is the portion size—probably double or triple what I recommend. So try to restrain yourself, even though it tastes so good, and eat only half of what is on your plate; bring the rest home in a doggie bag.

There will be times, of course, when the day's special sounds just too enticing. Or you are on vacation and wish to be completely hedonistic. Or you've been invited to a dinner party and do not want to make a fuss or hurt the cook's feelings. As I've said before, with Dr. Rau's Way, you cannot cheat. If you've gone through detox and maintained a healthy diet after that for at least a month or two, eating whatever you like on occasion will not make any difference to your health. We are not designed to have to be perfect.

On the other hand, your body will tell you when you've indulged too often. If your business trip involves three meals out a day or you're on an extended vacation and simply want to eat everything you see while you're away, your body will let you know when it's gone too far. You'll feel it in your gut, your sinuses, your energy level, your mood. Whichever is your weak point. Or it could be just a feeling of malaise and mild depression.

When you feel you've gone too far, don't give up. Simply put yourself on my One-Week Intensive Cure, preferably coupled with our excellent Liver Cleanse, and you will feel like your better self again. After those seven days, you can go right back on the Maintenance Diet, though it's best to eat lightly the first few days after the cure.

CHAPTER NINE

The Holistic Pantry

CHANGING THE WAY YOU EAT

Once you've spent a couple of months on my Maintenance Diet for Life, eating to support your health will be second nature. You'll be enjoying the way you eat as much as the way you feel, you'll wonder why it took so long to find a better way. But getting started on anything new, especially a diet, can be difficult.

What many of my patients have found, especially the ones who are sophisticated about food and who enjoy dining out, is that the nutritional plan becomes much easier if you approach each meal as a culinary adventure. Think of switching over to this healthy way of eating the same way as renovating your kitchen. Except that instead of changing the look and color of the appliances and cabinets, you are remodeling the ingredients in your pantry and in your refrigerator.

There is one appliance I recommend you throw out right away: the microwave oven. The radiation is toxic and can cause cataracts and worse if there is any leakage from around the seals. Most good cooks have learned that it is good for little other than reheating, anyway, and that can be done quickly and efficiently on top of the stove. And while you're at it, toss out all those nonstick pans. When hot, the fumes cause sudden death in parrots. What do you think they're doing to *your* lungs?

Treat yourself instead to a really good large stainless-steel saucepan and lid with a steamer insert or an inexpensive Chinese bamboo steamer. It will make meal preparation quick and your life very easy.

Following a sensible nutritional plan does not mean depriving yourself of the pleasures of dining. Once you're past detox, being able to make choices about what you eat, indulge a whim, or satisfy a craving for a particular food can be liberating. What's important is making the right choices.

Whether you're doing the Swiss Detox Diet or my Maintenance Diet for Life, you'll be eating many vegetables—steamed, poached, and roasted. So you'll want to stock up on a variety of produce, especially carrots, potatoes, beets, and broccoli and leafy greens. It's nice to vary the colors and textures on your plate while getting all the valuable nutrients you need. Look for heirloom varieties, which often have delightful variations of color and flavor. Having a large stock of ingredients to choose from makes throwing together salads or designing a plate of steamed vegetables much easier. As with your health, you'll feel better about anything you do if you are empowered to make your own choices.

For some reason, people think that when you eat mostly vegetables, it's monotonous. But the many recipes you'll find in this book will prove anything but dull. A huge selection not only of fruits and vegetables but of whole grains, free-range chicken, and healthy fish should round out your meals nicely.

Once you've entered the maintenance stage and are eating for your health for the rest of your life, finding the best of the foods that are good for you becomes all the more important. That's why I recommend shopping at a very good supermarket or specialty food store that stocks a wide assortment of organic produce and what used to be called health food ingredients. In summer, find an organic vegetable farm near you, and look for local growers and farmers who raise their animals naturally and can supply you with other wholesome ingredients.

If you like to cook, having a wide range of foods available will ensure you don't feel deprived of creativity. If you don't enjoy cooking, it will still afford you the pleasure of planning a variety of meals. Given the number of vegetarian cookbooks published each year, many of them bestsellers, Dr. Rau's Way hardly proposes anything outlandish or overly strict. But you must pay attention, because not all diets are alike, and my way is unique.

As with any other kind of cooking, the shopping is half the battle. Once you have the ingredients you need in the house, you'll be ready to go. And very quickly you'll discover that once you give up certain highly perishable items, especially cow's milk, fresh meat, and shellfish, shopping is a lot easier.

Many of the staples of Dr. Rau's Way, such as cereals and whole grains, can be banked away in the cupboard. Root vegetables—such as beets, carrots, potatoes, and parsnips—keep well for at least a couple of weeks. And the organic fresh vegetables and fruits that provide the base of the diet are easy to pick up once or twice a week at a local greengrocer.

Make Way for Good Nutrition

First of all, clean out your pantry. Get rid of everything that is totally forbidden, both to make room for the healthy foods you are going to purchase and to remove temptation.

Remove from Your Cupboards

- White flour

- White sugar

- White flour crackers, especially those containing trans fats (which are what make them crisp)

- Cookies and coffee cakes

- Fried tortilla chips

- Canned and bottled juices and sodas

- Processed foods, which are loaded with preservatives, sodium, sugar, eggs, dried milk, and trans fats (when in doubt, read the labels)
  - Pancake mix
  - Dehydrated foods, such as stuffings and helpers
  - Products containing genetically modified foods, such as many brands of soy protein flakes
  - Candy, especially milk chocolate
  - Commercial peanut butter
  - Evaporated or condensed cow's milk
  - Bread crumbs, like panko, which contain preservatives and trans fats
  - Commercial salsas
  - Seasonings that have monosodium glutamate (MSG), which is also called hydrolyzed vegetable protein
  - Canned fruits and vegetables

Remove from the Refrigerator and Freezer

- All chicken, turkey, lamb, and beef that is not labeled organic

- All pork and pork products, period, including bacon

- Frozen farmed salmon, swordfish, or other large bottom-feeding fish, like monkfish

- Shrimp

- Mayonnaise

- Jams, jellies, and pickles

- Cured meats or fish

- Commercial ketchup, which is loaded with sugar

- All cow's milk products, whether they are organic or not: milk, half-and-half, yogurt, cottage cheese, cream cheese, ice cream, Cheddar cheese, and any other cheeses make from cow's milk, even if they are artisanally produced. And, yes, sadly that includes Parmesan cheese, though many people can tolerate a little bit of imported Parmigiano Reggiano once in a while. Assuming you don't have high cholesterol, a little bit of butter or heavy cream is okay, especially because there will be so little saturated fat in the rest of your diet.

Check Out Your Vegetable Bin

Unless you live in a region where you absolutely cannot obtain organic fruits and vegetables, add all that inorganic produce to your compost heap. One of my patients who lives in a very rural area grows some of her own vegetables in season and buys the rest from a local organic farm; in winter, she orders her organic produce by mail order. They arrive in a box once a week via a ground shipping service.

Throw out your onions and shallots. I know they add flavor to food, but they also thicken lymphatic fluids. Leeks are a milder allium that do contribute a fine aromatic quality to foods and are permitted in small amounts. Use the white for cooking, the dark green for stocks, and the pale green part raw for salad, like Swiss Potato Salad (page 224). Garlic, too, can be used very sparingly, as can minced fresh chives.

Stock Up with the Right Foods

By now you should have plenty of extra room in your kitchen. It's time to start filling up those empty shelves with healthy foods that will keep your internal environment in perfect balance.

You probably won't have to go far. If you live in a city, you may make a few stops—at the greengrocer's, the butcher's, the health-food store. In most suburbs and now even in cities, there are now one-stop shopping superstores of all sorts that have large organic produce departments and aisles and aisles of foods that are good for you.

Bring your reading glasses, though, because you're really going to have to study labels carefully. A package of plain rye crisps, for example, which are an excellent choice for spreads and cheeses, contains nothing but rye flour and water. But a flavored version of the same brand may contain any number of additives, preservatives, and even trans fats you don't want.

There's an irony that while the population of America in general is getting fatter and fatter (almost two thirds of the U.S. population is clinically overweight and more than a third are morbidly obese) and type 2 diabetes is growing in epidemic proportions, upscale supermarkets tempt their customers with beautiful fruits and vegetables. When you first enter the store, it's the gorgeous fruits and vegetables that are displayed up front. That's wonderful—just what you need. But take a good look, and make sure the aisle you are in is filled with organics.

In days gone by, *organic* was just a word thrown around casually. Not long ago, however, it was responsibly adopted into law in the United States, so that when you see a label that says "certified organic"—whether on a chicken or a vegetable—it really means something. It is a symbol of quality in terms of nutritional health. And as mentioned in the previous chapter, it indicates that that fruit or vegetable—or chicken—will taste better, too.

Once you reach my Maintenance Diet for Life, you are allowed small servings of chicken and fish two or three times a week, and even beef or lamb once in a while, if you really feel you need them. But all these meats should be organic, raised on vegetable feed with no antibiotics or hormones, so if what you have in the freezer doesn't meet these standards, get rid of it. Expensive, I know, but isn't your health worth every penny? Even ordinary supermarkets these days often sell more than one brand of

WHAT DOES "CERTIFIED ORGANIC" REALLY MEAN?

"Certified organic" is a legal term established by the U.S. Department of Agriculture (USDA). It is a label that asserts fruits, vegetables, and other agricultural products have been grown and processed according to the USDA's national organic standards. Certification is a stringent process that requires annual on-site inspection of farms, farmers, and processors by state and/or private USDA-accredited organizations that review how the land was used in the past and how it is being used in the present. The idea is to prevent the use of all artificial pesticides and toxic chemicals in the growing of produce and to ensure outdoor access (free range) for animals. In addition, agents make sure that the feed for organically raised animals is all-vegetable and free of antibiotics and hormones.

organic chicken. And natural meats are in upscale markets and easily obtainable by mail order. Look, too, to local farmers, who may well have much more humane ways of raising their animals than do large commercial establishments and factory farms.

Stock up, if necessary, so that the food is there when you want it, but when you are freezing meat, chicken, turkey, and fish, keep portion control in mind. When I say, assuming you are not extremely ill, you can have a little chicken or fish several times a week, I mean literally *a little:* a 3- to four-ounce portion is more than enough. So keep this mind when you are wrapping up cuts for freezing or even when you're planning what to cook. If you really feel like roast chicken on Sunday night, that would be lovely, assuming it is accompanied by plenty of vegetables, as well. But make sure you have enough people around the table to finish off most of that bird, because leftovers can be seductive and two days of chicken can easily stretch into three.

If you read half a dozen acid/alkaline diet books, you'll come away completely confused. There are at least six different lists of which vegetables you can and cannot eat. Some macrobiotic books get in the game,

HOW TO SPROUT LENTILS

Sprouts are the most active, nutritionally vital forms of any vegetable. Also, in their sprouted state, lentils—as well as many other beans and seeds—are digestible even though technically raw so that none of the nutrition is lost in the heat of cooking. Lentils are easy to sprout and very palatable; mung beans also sprout well as do some seeds, such as alfalfa. Just a tablespoon or two is a very nice, healthful addition to any salad.

You can use a loosely covered plastic storage container lined with a damp paper towel, but sprouters just for this purpose are inexpensive and easy to find in health-food stores and on the Internet. They usually have grooves for the moisture to drain off, so the lentils don't get moldy.

Simply rinse the lentils well. Without drying them, spread out in a single layer in the sprouter. Cover and set aside in a warm place with light. Sprouting takes anywhere from 12 to 48 hours, depending on the temperature. As soon as they sprout, transfer the lentils to a covered container and refrigerate. Use within three days. You can sprout almost any seed in similar fashion.

as well, providing laundry lists of what one can and cannot eat based on no known form of science. One book will claim that avocados are acidic, another that zucchini is taboo. To be blunt, this is ridiculous. With the exception of a few vegetables and fruits like oranges that are very high in sugar, which makes them acidic, your body will metabolize most fruits and vegetables as alkaline, and they are all excellent for your health.

What may be a little confusing is that some fruits we think of as acidic, such as lemons and grapefruits, actually metabolize as alkaline. So please relax and enjoy the variety from your garden, greengrocer, or organic section of your supermarket. Just so you feel comfortable, here is a list of all the produce you can enjoy as well as other foods you'll want to stock up on.

FRUITS

apples	grapefruit	pineapple
apricots	grapes	plums
bananas	lemons	prunes
blueberries	mangoes	raisins
cantaloupe	melon	raspberries
cherries	papayas	strawberries
currants	peaches	watermelon
dates	pears	

VEGETABLES

When it comes to vegetables, the list of all the good foods you can enjoy is even longer. Many fibrous vegetables are best eaten shredded if raw. Otherwise, your body cannot break them down. At the same time, the slow digestion of raw vegetables keeps your blood sugar comfortably elevated and very stable. You can shred most vegetables on the large holes of a box grater or—much easier—on the shredding/grating disk of your food processor. For softer vegetables, like zucchini, the julienne disk works better to cut finely without mashing.

While many good cooks were trained to blanch vegetables in a large pot of boiling water, steaming not only locks in more color, flavor, and nutrients, it is quicker. Roasting is another way of intensifying flavor.

artichoke	broccoli rabe
arugula	cabbage
asparagus	carrots
avocado	cauliflower
beans and other legumes	celery
(once a week as a main dish,	celery root (celeriac)
in small amounts as you like)	collard greens
beets	corn
bell peppers (in small amounts)	cucumbers
bok choy	daikon
broccoli	eggplant

endive

escarole

fresh fennel (anise)

ginger

green beans

jicama

kale

kohlrabi

leeks (only a little)

lentils

lettuce

mushrooms (in small amounts)

mustard greens

parsnips

peas

pea shoots

potatoes

pumpkin

radishes

Romanesco (broccoflower)

sauerkraut, especially
    homemade

seaweed

soy (in small amounts)

spinach

sprouts

squash

Swiss chard

tofu (in small amounts)

tomato (only when homegrown
    or organic, in season)

turnip

watercress

zucchini

NUTS AND SEEDS

Many people are allergic to some nuts, like hazelnuts, walnuts, and peanuts. That's why they are not on this list. However, many of these allergies seem to be generational. If you believe you are *not* allergic to peanuts or another nut, do the Maintenance test: Eat a little at one meal and pay close attention for several days to see if you notice any symptoms. If not, repeat. When you know you're home free, add that nut to your list of acceptable foods. Remember, a great deal of this diet is individual. Seeds, too, are an important source of nutrients in a largely vegetarian diet.

almonds (in small amounts;
    only if you are not allergic)

cashews

chestnuts

coconuts

flax seeds

macadamia nuts

pecans

pine nuts	sesame seeds
pumpkin seeds	sunflower seeds

SWEETENERS

White sugar, which is processed with arsenic, is completely forbidden. All sweeteners should be used minimally, because they are acidic. There are other forms of sweeteners, such as stevia and agave, which some vegetarians use, but all the recipes in this book call for ingredients with which you are already familiar:

Raw sugar

Maple syrup—Amber has the most flavor

Honey—Excellent organic honeys abound. Choose a mild one, such as wildflower or linden, and a deeper-flavored honey, such as chestnut.

OTHER PANTRY ITEMS

Natural sea salt or Himalayan salt

Herbs and spices. Unless you are allergic, all are permitted with the exception of fresh cilantro and dried coriander, which are the same plant—many people have a reaction to this herb. If you don't think you are allergic, do the test before eating in quantity.

Organic vegetable bouillon powder (makes many vegetarian dishes easy to prepare, with fewer ingredients; choose a brand that contains no MSG)

Organic vegetable and chicken stock

Rice milk	Arborio rice
Rice crackers	Basmati rice
Rye crisps	Extra virgin olive oil
Rice noodles	Sunflower oil
Soy milk	Asian sesame oil
Spelt pasta	Pumpkin seed oil
Buckwheat pasta	Balsamic vinegar
Imported semolina pasta	Rice vinegar

CHAPTER TEN

Dr. Rau's One-Week Intensive Cure

WHEN YOU NEED A QUICK FIX

As I often say, with Dr. Rau's Way you cannot cheat. That means if you feel like a steak once in a while and all the rest of the time you follow my diet, it will not make a bit of difference. (Although I always hope that if my patients indulge in a protein fix, it's a small portion.) If you've gone through the three-week detox and you've been on my Maintenance Diet for Life for at least a couple of months, you have already altered your internal environment much for the better: you've made over your intestinal flora, calmed your primary food allergies, alkalized your system, and bolstered your immune system. Your body is resilient, and one steak or a slice of chocolate cake is not going to make any difference to your well-being.

However, if bad nutrition becomes a habit, over time it's going to take a toll. Say you've been on the road for work or away on vacation, and you've indulged in rich restaurant food every night, eating whatever you wanted. Or you've been down in the dumps and comforting yourself with hamburgers and fries or ice cream and pie. Perhaps you have a substance dependency, and you've slipped. At some point, you will have gone too far. You only have so much leeway before your system tips out of balance.

You won't need anyone to tell you when you've overindulged: your body will let you know when it's had enough. Perhaps you'll get a little depressed. Maybe your sinuses will act up. Your digestion may start giving you trouble. Your sleep may be disturbed. You may put on a lot of weight all at once. Or you may just feel terrible.

Of course, to clean out again, you can always return to the Swiss Detox Diet, but that's a three-week program. For those who have already gone through nutritional detox and have for some time at least maintained their body in regulatory balance, I offer this quick fix: Dr. Rau's One-Week Intensive Cure. It's a seven-day cleansing diet that carries enough punch to bring you back to go. And it's especially effective when combined with our excellent Liver Cleanse, which you'll find in the next chapter. This opens up the bile ducts and cleans out old congested fats from the liver and gallbladder. Many of our longtime patients revisit the Paracelsus Clinic or our sister clinic Al Ronc in the Alps once a year for a weeklong refresher cleanse that pairs this diet with the Liver Cleanse.

In lieu of a fast, which can be both damaging and counterproductive, I developed this cleansing diet, which lasts for seven days. It consists of just enough food to maintain healthy electrolyte balance and to stimulate your digestive juices so that old toxic proteins are burned up and passed out. It also speeds up cellular metabolism, which results in faster detoxification and weight loss.

You could almost view this week as a purge. The nutritional program consists of a highly restricted vegetarian diet—in terms of both foods and amounts—that cleanses the liver, kidneys, and other organs, efficiently flushing out toxins from the body in a short amount of time. In fact, if you'll pardon my frankness, when you stop forcing food in one end, the toxins start coming out the other. At our clinics in Switzerland, this diet is accompanied by colonics and other treatments. At home, enemas can achieve much of the same benefit, though, of course, they are not as thorough.

Drinking large amounts of water—at least 2 to 3 liters a day—is mandatory to flush out your system and maintain equilibrium. We also suggest herbal teas, such as lime blossom and rosemary, which increase metabolism. Whatever the state of your health, this potent diet is rejuvenating as well as excellent for weight loss. Many people are surprised at how refreshed they feel after only seven days. That's because this program actually has all the detoxifying and stimulating benefits of a liquid fast without the detrimental rebound effect most people suffer afterward. Let me explain.

I noticed this syndrome early in my career, when I was in charge of rehabilitation at a large hospital. Fasting is a common cure in Europe, and many patients who came for long-term care would begin their treatment with a weeklong fast, depriving themselves of all solid food and drinking only water and a little fruit juice. After the fast, most of the patients felt much better—no matter what illness or symptoms they were suffering from when they arrived.

This made sense, because without realizing what they were doing, they were avoiding foods they were allergic to, not ingesting any new toxins or pollutants, and staying away from protein, which allowed some of the old toxins built up in their body to be expressed, thus preparing their systems for healing. However, the very next week, I noticed that the same patients were much worse than they were originally—their symptoms were aggravated to an extreme.

Finally, I put it together and realized what the problem was. On a complete fast, cells begin to detoxify, working loose old toxins and degraded proteins, even some heavy metals. But because the body is taking in little or no nutrients, it is tricked into thinking it is sick or about to be starved, so it goes into retentive mode. That's part of the wonderful resilience of human beings. If you are starving or too ill to eat, your body shifts gears, as it were, so it can operate on a lower metabolic level and conserve all its energy and resources to survive. It holds on to everything. (This is also why people on too strict a weight-loss diet lose dramatically at first but then quickly regain each pound, sometimes even adding a few extra.)

Unfortunately, for those fasting patients, the toxins that blocked their systems were shaken loose to a certain extent. But because their bodies were shocked into retentive mode by the complete fast, the toxins remained stuck within. The patients' bodies could not let go of them, and the harmful toxins came back at them with even greater force. In addition, when the body is starving, it begins to reduce all nonessential metabolic functions. The organism holds back and saves everything it can. Even pituitary and adrenal functions are lowered, which is counterproductive.

This is why my One-Week Intensive Cure is designed to simulate the benefits of a complete fast while forcing the body into a releasing, or purging, mode instead. By tricking the body—that is, keeping it supplied with what it needs to stimulate cell metabolism—the detoxification is quick and powerful.

As I said, think of this week as a quick fix. It's not normally necessary, but it's there if you need it. I say you can't cheat, but if you stray too much or too often, eventually your body's balance will be compromised. When that happens, you don't need to worry about it; just do something about it. One week, and you can return to Maintenance.

Aside from cheating, other life events can throw us off balance. Even if you're essentially well and you've been following my Maintenance Diet for some time, you may go through a difficult patch. Injuries occur, family stresses arise, work pressure can undermine otherwise good habits. From time to time we all feel like we need a boost. And that's just what this week offers.

If you're suffering from specific symptoms, you may be surprised at how fast they begin to subside. Because whether you feel sluggish and depressed; have a host of vague symptoms; suffer from an intractable problem like chronic headaches, indigestion, or undefined pain; or already have a diagnosis of a serious illness, the basis of all health is the same: an optimally functioning body is a well-regulated body in metabolic balance.

Step-by-step instructions for the seven-day cure are given later in this chapter. By greatly restricting your caloric and nutritional intake while flushing out your system with a large amount of fluid and purging at the same time, you punch a big hole in that barrel and get rid of many toxins.

Seven Days to Better Health

If you are ready for my One-Week Intensive Cure, here's how it works. For one week you follow a strict vegetarian diet with small amounts of food and plenty of appropriate liquids: vegetable broth, fresh vegetable juices, herbal teas, and pure spring water. I know some health–conscious people like to fast completely from time to time, but a strict fast with no food at all is actually very stressful on your body. What's worse, as ex- plained earlier, it is counterproductive. Deprived of all nutrition, your body seizes up and goes into starvation mode. Your metabolism slows down, and your body holds on to as much of its stored material as it can. It actually makes it harder to purge. That's not what we want.

Our goal is to do the opposite, to trick the body into opening up and releasing excessive and degraded toxic proteins and fatty deposits. With the One-Week Intensive Cure, your metabolism will actually speed up, causing a corresponding release of large amounts of toxins and poisons, rather than the retention caused by fasting. Ironically, because of this, you'll actually lose more weight than on a total fast.

During the intensive cure, small amounts of light foods are eaten at crit- ical times, often enough to prevent your blood sugar from crashing. You must chew each bite 20 to 30 times. Not only does this give you the sensa- tion of eating more, it stimulates the digestive juices to encourage digestion and elimination of all the old, excess proteins that have been clogging up your body for years. This purge forces them out of the tissues to the lymph and blood to where they can be processed by the liver. Especially if you are sick, it is important to detoxify with control, so that your body can remain strong and begin improving your internal environment at once.

At the same time, purging is encouraged to further eliminate toxic substances and cleanse the intestines. Only by rinsing out all the bad bacteria and old detritus, by laying out a clean healthy soil, as it were, can you encourage the growth of good bacteria, upon which the health of your entire immune system is built.

This internal cleansing is very important. At the Paracelsus Clinic, we give patients high colonics of a very particular sort. They are accompanied by a gentle massaging of the abdomen, which stimulates the parasympathetic nervous system, stimulating your intestines to function better. This helps the body to let go, pushing out waste from high up without risking too much intrusion. These colonics rid the body of toxins that collect in the intestines, old putrid matter, and damaging intestinal bacteria. At the clinic, these cleansings are followed immediately by a replanting, so to speak, of a specific intestinal flora, the kind that is so important for the digestion and absorption of all nutrients. The result is that one system at least is completely cleaned out, toned up, and ready to go.

At home, you can achieve some of the same effect by taking a warm-water or mild organic coffee enema on the evening of your second day on the Intensive Cure and a second on the evening of the sixth day. Alternatively, on days two and six, first thing in the morning, drink 1 tablespoon Epsom salts dissolved in 1 cup warm water to encourage elimination.

As I noted, the One-Week Intensive Cure is most effective when combined with our Liver Cleanse, which you'll find in the next chapter. The two go hand in hand to provide the best results in the shortest amount of time. If you are doing the Liver Cleanse, which I hope you will do, you must also drink at least 1 liter of apple juice each day to open up the bile ducts.

Liquids Are Extremely Important

Because so much waste is being expelled from the body, you must be absolutely rigorous about drinking enough fluids to flush out the kidneys, prevent dehydration, and maintain your electrolyte balance. At least 2½ to 3 liters (about 2½ to 3 quarts) of liquid a day is recommended.

These liquids should include the following:

Vegetable Juices

Each day 4 ounces (½ cup) fresh vegetable juice is prescribed. Beet and carrot juices are especially good for you, but almost any vegetable is appropriate. People with delicate stomachs respond well to 1 to 2 tablespoons of raw potato juice, which is excellent for "leaky gut syndrome." All vegetables must be organic to avoid more toxic load from pesticides and fertilizers. If you own a juicer, freshly squeezed is best. Or maybe you have a juice store near you. If not, look for a good organic brand in your local health-food store. The vegetable juice is best drunk as a cocktail at dinner.

Fruit Juices

A small (4-ounce) glass of grapefruit juice, preferably pink, should be taken in the morning. Unsweetened apple juice, preferably the European kind, which is much more like our fresh cider, is essential if you will be doing the Liver Cleanse. Drink at least 1 liter a day, sipping it slowly in between meals.

Herbal Teas

You can enjoy 4 cups or more of herb teas. Certain herbal teas tend to stimulate elimination. We particularly recommend fennel tea, stinging nettle tea, linden blossom tea, and peppermint tea, as well as wormwood tea, if you can get it. These particular varieties stimulate the metabolism. No sweetener is allowed.

Vegetable Broth

Dr. Rau's Alkaline Soup (page 152) is easy to make, and one batch will last for two days. You will enjoy 2½ to 3 cups of this each day, but no salt—not even sea salt—is allowed. Be sure not to include any of the vegetables from the soup unless stipulated by the diet, which is outlined later in the chapter. Dr. Rau's broth can be sipped throughout the day, if you wish.

Water

At least 1 liter of your fluids should be nonchlorinated, noncarbonated spring water, preferably purified, with as few minerals as possible. Drink all water at room temperature or warmer. No chilled or iced drinks.

In addition, twice a day, at 10:00 A.M. and 4:00 P.M., you should drink ½ measuring spoon of Alkala, which is found in many health-food stores, or about ½ teaspoon of another alkalizing powder, such as bicarbonate of soda, dissolved in half a glass of warm water. This also encourages elimination.

Despite all the fluids you are drinking, over the course of the week, most people lose 4 to 5 pounds of weight. Best of all, when it is all over you will look and feel marvelous.

What to Expect When You Cleanse

A strenuous week of purging like this is best undertaken with the least amount of stress possible. That's why people often visit a retreat or a spa to detoxify. If you can, make this a quiet week. Many patients come to our clinic, which faces the rolling meadows and far mountains of the Appenzell, or to Al Ronc, perched on the side of the Alps near the Italian border, for a relaxing week of detox combined with our powerful Liver Cleanse. Resting in a chaise lounge set out on a sunny terrace facing the glorious snow-covered Alps certainly helps reduce stress. We also offer all kinds of therapeutic and relaxing treatments.

You can go to work and function perfectly well if you need to during this time, but do try to maintain a low stress level. Keep early hours and cut back on your ordinary fitness program, if you have one. You might consider scheduling a massage. Take plenty of relaxing baths and hot showers. If you do yoga or meditate, concentrate on those excellent methods of relieving stress and stimulating your parasympathetic (unconscious) nervous system. A half-hour walk once or twice a day will always do you good, but stay away from the gym. Don't over-exert yourself. You want to be as kind to your body as possible during this period, so it can do its important work. Let go as much as you can. Try to make it a peaceful week. You are turning your mind around along with your body.

If possible, take the week off from work. If you have a country home, take advantage of it. If you stay home, unplug the phone, leave the television off, don't read the newspaper. Surround yourself with beautiful objects, flowers, plants, or sounds that please you. Strive for serenity.

The Intensive Cure can be a very intimate experience to share with a partner. Because you are retreating from many of the usual distractions and focusing inward, many couples find they often bind closely during this week.

This is an appropriate time to allow your spiritual life to manifest itself. Leave your computer at the office. Take advantage of this extra time to think about yourself and your life. What is really most important? Your health, to be sure. And your loved ones. If you have a serious or chronic illness, this is a good time to examine your life. Are your priorities in order? Are you making the right choices in your life? Are there stresses you can relieve without making any major changes? Surely, we all have much to think about and rarely a week like this in which to do it.

Getting Ready for the Cure

On a practical level, get all the physical arrangements you can out of the way in the beginning. Plan what foods you need and do your shopping ahead of time. No restaurants or gourmet markets this week. Most of what you require is an appetizing selection of beautiful organic vegetables and a few healthy whole grains that contain no gluten: quinoa, amaranth, millet, buckwheat, and cornmeal. You'll need fresh vegetable juices, gallons of purified spring water, some apples and lots of unsweetened apple juice, and a selection of herb teas. Decide if you are going to handle food preparation, minimal as it is, or if someone is going to help you. You will need to make a batch of Dr. Rau's Alkaline Soup every other day. Try not to think about indulgences like fine food and wine. At this point, think only of your liver, glutted with fat and bulging with toxins.

The one recipe you will definitely need to prepare is my cleansing Dr. Rau's Alkaline Soup. It's utterly simple to make and has only four main ingredients; but it will sustain you well. The broth is taken first thing in the morning and at dinner. You can have another cup at lunch, if you wish. At dinner, more of the broth is served along with a little bit of the vegetables from the soup, mashed into a puree.

Dr. Rau's Alkaline Soup
■ MAKES ABOUT 7 CUPS BROTH; 3½ CUPS VEGETABLES

1½ cups finely diced (⅜-inch) zucchini

1 cup thinly cut green beans (about 4 ounces)

¾ cup finely diced (¼- to ⅛-inch) celery root or 2 celery ribs, finely diced

¾ cup finely diced (¼- to ⅛-inch) peeled carrots

Sea salt (optional)

1. Put all the vegetables in a large saucepan with 2 quarts of pure (nonchlorinated) spring water. Bring to a boil; skim off any scum that rises to the top.
2. Reduce the heat to a simmer, partially cover the pot, and cook the vegetables for 10 to 12 minutes, or until they are soft.
3. Remove from the heat and let stand, covered, for 10 minutes. Serve as directed. Once you move on to the Maintenance Diet for Life, you may season the broth with salt to taste.

NOTE: If you wish to double, or even triple, the recipe so you have a good stock of alkalizing broth on hand, you may do so, keeping only enough for two days in the refrigerator and freezing the rest in measured containers. However, the vegetables cannot be frozen and may only be eaten the first two days; any leftovers must be discarded.

Now that you have made all your arrangements and prepared my alkaline soup, you are all ready to go. Here are the basics for the One-Week Intensive Cure:

- No meat
- No sugar
- No gluten
- No dairy
- No nuts (except for chestnuts)
- No salt or pepper
- At least 3 liters of fluids a day, including pure spring water, broth from Dr. Rau's Alkaline Soup, vegetable juices, herbal teas, and unsweetened organic apple juice, if you are doing the Liver Cleanse

Although you are prescribed three meals a day plus two small snacks to maintain your blood sugar, the food is very light in quantity and substance and heavy on the vegetables. So to digest it properly and to make yourself feel as satisfied as possible, be sure to chew each bite 20 to 30 times. You absolutely *must* drink all your fluids—at least 3 liters—both to hydrate yourself and especially to flush out all the toxins that will be surfacing. Keep a relaxed schedule and go to bed early. Supper should be eaten no later than 6:30, if at all possible. And if you are doing the Liver Cleanse, be sure to drink at least 1 liter of unsweetened apple juice in addition to the other liquids.

DAY 1

Breakfast

- 4 ounces (½ cup) fresh grapefruit juice, preferably Ruby Red **or** pink

- 1 cup broth (no vegetables) from Dr. Rau's Alkaline Soup (page 152)

- ½ cup quinoa porridge, served with 2 halves of Poached Plums (page 297) and ⅓ cup plum poaching liquid

- 1 tablespoon pure flax seed oil

- ½ apple

- Cup of herb tea

Midmorning Snack

- ½ apple

Lunch

- SALAD PLATE: ½ cup loosely packed baby spinach leaves, ¼ cup shredded zucchini, and ¼ cup shredded carrots dressed with 1½ teaspoons each extra virgin olive oil and balsamic vinegar. No salt **or** pepper

- STEAMED VEGETABLE PLATE: ½ cup broccoli florets, ½ cup coarsely cut-up Swiss chard leaves, and ⅓ cup cut-up green beans dressed with 1½ teaspoons each extra virgin olive oil and fresh lemon juice

- Cup of herb tea

Midafternoon Snack

- ½ avocado with a squeeze of lemon juice

Supper

- 4 ounces (½ cup) fresh beet juice

- 1½ cups Dr. Rau's Alkaline Soup, with ⅓ cup vegetables from the soup

- STEAMED VEGETABLE PLATE: ½ small fennel bulb, thickly sliced, 4 asparagus spears, and ½ cup cauliflower florets dressed with 1½ teaspoons each extra virgin olive oil and fresh lemon juice

- 3 small rice crackers

- Cup of herb tea

DAY 2

Breakfast

- 4 ounces (½ cup) fresh grapefruit juice

- 1 cup broth (no vegetables) from Dr. Rau's Alkaline Soup

- ½ cup millet porridge, prepared with 2 teaspoons raisins, served with ½ cup rice milk

- 1 tablespoon pure flax seed oil

- ½ apple

- Cup of herb tea

Midmorning Snack

- ½ small avocado with a squeeze of lemon juice

Lunch

- SALAD PLATE: 1 cup loosely packed baby field greens, ¼ cup shredded carrot, ¼ cup shredded raw beet, and 2 radishes thinly sliced, dressed with 1½ teaspoons each extra virgin olive oil and balsamic vinegar

■ STEAMED VEGETABLE PLATE: ⅓ cup halved sugarsnap peas, ½ cup broccoli florets, and 1 cup loosely packed spinach leaves (before cooking), dressed with 1½ teaspoons each extra virgin olive oil and fresh lemon juice

■ Cup of herb tea

Midafternoon Snack

■ ½ apple

Supper

■ 4 ounces (½ cup) fresh carrot juice

■ 1½ cups Sweet Corn and Potato Chowder (page 202), made with no butter, and omitting the salt and pepper

■ STEAMED VEGETABLE PLATE: ⅓ cup cut-up green beans, 2 thick slices of kohlrabi **or** celery root, and 1 cup (loosely packed before cooking) cut-up Swiss chard stem and leaves, dressed with 1½ teaspoons each extra virgin olive oil and fresh lemon juice

■ Cup of herb tea

DAY 3

Breakfast

■ 4 ounces (½ cup) fresh grapefruit juice

■ 1 cup broth (no vegetables) from Dr. Rau's Alkaline Soup

■ ⅔ cup unsweetened amaranth cereal, served with ½ sliced small banana and ½ cup rice milk

■ 1 tablespoon pure flax seed oil

■ ½ apple

■ Cup of herb tea

Midmorning Snack

- 1 small carrot

Lunch

- SALAD PLATE: ⅓ cup Corn, Rice, and Pea Salad (page 220), 1 cup loosely packed baby spinach leaves, and ⅓ cup shredded zucchini dressed with 1½ teaspoons each extra virgin olive oil and fresh lemon juice

- STEAMED VEGETABLE PLATE: ½ yellow summer squash, sliced, and 1 cup (loosely packed before cooking) shredded kale dressed with 1½ teaspoons each extra virgin olive oil and balsamic vinegar and served with ⅓ cup Marinated Roasted Beets (page 219)

- Cup of herb tea

Midafternoon Snack

- 4 cooked chestnuts

Supper

- 4 ounces (½ cup) zucchini and celery juice

- 1½ cups Dr. Rau's Alkaline Soup, including ½ cup diced vegetables from the soup

- Fennel Gratin (omitting the cheese) (page 244)

- Cup of herb tea

DAY 4

Breakfast

- Same as Day 1

Midmorning Snack

- ½ avocado with a squeeze of lemon juice

Lunch

- SALAD PLATE: ⅔ cup loosely packed baby arugula, ⅓ cup thinly sliced cucumber, ⅓ cup sliced celery, and 2 radishes, thinly sliced, dressed with 1½ teaspoons each extra virgin olive oil and balsamic vinegar

- STEAMED VEGETABLE PLATE: ⅓ cup baby peas, ⅔ cup broccoli florets, and 1 small fennel bulb, quartered, dressed with 1½ teaspoons each extra virgin olive oil and fresh lemon juice

Midafternoon Snack

- 1 small carrot

Supper

- 4 ounces (½ cup) fresh beet juice

- 1½ cups Dr. Rau's Alkaline Soup, including ½ cup diced vegetables from the soup

- Asparagus Stir-Fry with Swiss Chard and Carrots (page 240), omitting the cashews. Serve with ¼ cup steamed basmati rice.

- Cup of herb tea

DAY 5

Breakfast

- Same as Day 2

Midmorning Snack

■ 1 small cucumber

Lunch

■ SALAD PLATE: 1 cup baby field greens and ⅓ cup shredded zucchini dressed with 1½ teaspoons each extra virgin olive oil and balsamic vinegar and served with ⅓ cup Shredded Beet and Carrot Salad (page 218) and ⅓ cup Swiss Potato Salad (page 224) made without any leek **or** salt and pepper

■ ½ portion Corn, Rice, and Pea Salad

■ Cup of herb tea

Midafternoon Snack

■ 5 small rice crackers

Supper

■ 4 ounces (½ cup) fresh carrot juice

■ 1½ cups Quick Broccoli Soup (page 198), omitting the cream and salt

■ STEAMED VEGETABLE PLATE: 6 asparagus spears, ½ small sweet potato, sliced, and 1 cup coarsely cut up (before cooking) broccoli rabe, dressed with 1½ teaspoons each extra virgin olive oil and fresh lemon juice

■ Cup of herb tea

DAY 6

Breakfast

■ 4 ounces (½ cup) fresh grapefruit juice

■ 1 cup broth (no vegetables) from Dr. Rau's Alkaline Soup

- ⅓ cup buckwheat groats cooked to a porridge with 1 cup water and no salt until soft, about 15 minutes

- 1 tablespoon pure flax seed oil

- ½ apple

- Cup of herb tea

Midmorning Snack

- ½ avocado, with a squeeze of fresh lemon juice

Lunch

- SALAD PLATE: 1 cup shredded romaine lettuce, ⅓ cup shredded carrots, ½ cup thinly sliced cucumber, and ⅓ cup bean sprouts, dressed with 1½ teaspoons each extra virgin olive oil and fresh lemon juice

- STEAMED VEGETABLE PLATE: 6 cooked chestnuts, ½ cup Marinated Roasted Beets (page 219), ½ cup cut-up green beans, and ½ small zucchini dressed with 1½ teaspoons each extra virgin olive oil and fresh lemon juice

- Cup of herb tea

Midafternoon Snack

- ½ small sweet potato, steamed

Supper

- 4 ounces (½ cup) mixed fresh beet and carrot juice flavored with fresh ginger

- 1½ cups Dr. Rau's Alkaline Soup with ½ cup diced vegetables from the soup

- ½ portion Sesame Quinoa with Bok Choy and Shiitake Mushrooms (page 242), omitting the mushrooms

- Cup of herb tea

DAY 7

Note: This is the day you will do your Liver Cleanse.

Breakfast

- Same as Day 3

Midmorning Snack

- 1 small apple

Lunch

- Same as Day 3

Supper

- If you're doing the Liver Cleanse, you should take nothing but liquids after 2:00 in the afternoon. If you're not, have a bowl of Dr. Rau's Alkaline Soup with ½ cup of the cooked vegetables from the soup and your choice of steamed vegetables. After dinner, have a cup of herb tea.

Now you must surely be totally refreshed, if perhaps a little hungry. If you are interested in weight loss, you will be pleased when you step on the scale. With so many toxins flushed from your system, you will look rejuvenated. Even in just a week, your connective tissue will strengthen, your skin will glow and appear tighter, and your eyes will look clearer. Most importantly, you will have undone any damage and can return to the Maintenance Diet for Life as if nothing ever happened.

CHAPTER ELEVEN

The Liver Cleanse

I highly recommend our powerful Liver Cleanse, which purifies both the liver and the gallbladder. It opens up the bile ducts, allowing excess fat and toxins to drain out in soft bilious stones. As I noted, this easy but extremely effective purge cleanses not only the liver but the gallbladder and bile ducts as well. And you can practice it in the privacy of your home, with little inconvenience. The only supplies you need are plenty of fresh organic lemons, 1 or 2 organic grapefruits (preferably Ruby Red or pink), Epsom salts, extra virgin olive oil, and gallons of unsweetened apple juice or fresh cider. (The only people who should not do the cleanse are pregnant and nursing mothers and anyone who is fructose intolerant.)

While the cleanse can be done at any time, it is by far best paired with the One-Week Intensive Cure, detailed in the previous chapter. That's because you must first prepare your body in very specific nutritional ways for about a week. Beginning at least seven days before the cleanse, you must abstain from all caffeine, alcohol, meat, cheese and other dairy, eggs, wheat, processed foods, and any other source of saturated fat. You should during this time eat a lot of shredded raw and lightly steamed vegetables, dressed only with lemon juice or balsamic vinegar and extra virgin olive oil. You may have natural sea salt or Himalayan salt and herbs, but no table salt: that is, sodium chloride. And most important for the cleanse, you must drink 1 to 2 liters of apple juice or cider between meals every day for at least 6 days. The malolactic acid in the apple juice opens up and relaxes the bile ducts and thins the bile so that the treatment is comfortable and completely painless.

I highly recommend the Liver Cleanse to anyone who has "fallen off the wagon," and wants to detoxify quickly so he or she can return to their ordinary Maintenance Diet for Life. In difficult times, it also offers a great way to jump-start your path to healing the Swiss biological medicine way. For you to understand why you might want to try the Liver Cleanse, it helps to understand how this amazing organ relates to your overall health.

About the Liver

The liver is the third largest organ in the body after the skin and the intestines. Situated on the right side of your upper abdomen, it is tucked in behind your diaphragm, right next to the stomach. Weighing anywhere from roughly 2½ to 3 pounds, the organ is absolutely vital to a slew of biochemical functions. If your liver stops working, you will die within 24 hours. One problem with chemotherapy—and even with many common pharmaceutical drugs, such as anti-inflammatories, statins, and antibiotics—is how much damage it does to the liver. The good news is that if given half a chance, the liver is extremely efficient at regenerating itself. And just about everything we do with Swiss biological medicine—especially the nutritional plan supported by Dr. Rau's Way—is dedicated to improving liver function.

What is extremely interesting about the liver is its dual nature: The organ is involved in both up-building—that is, construction of substances your body requires—and in degeneration—elimination of toxins and dead cells. It is both a complex chemical factory and a great detoxifying filtering machine.

Among the many chemicals the liver produces are bile and cholesterol. Bile, a digestive acid, is stored in the reservoir of the gallbladder, which then releases it into the small intestine as needed when you eat. Bile is essential for the digestion of fats and the absorption of fat-soluble vitamins. You cannot digest fat without bile, which is why people with gallbladder problems have to be so careful about what they eat. At the same time, it should be noted that many supposed gallbladder problems actually arise in the liver.

The liver also manufactures cholesterol. Despite all the bad publicity cholesterol in general gets, high-density lipoprotein (HDL) is an extremely important substance for forming cell walls, making many hormones, and cleaning up the bad low-density lipoprotein (LDL) in your bloodstream. About 60 percent of your brain is composed of fat containing cholesterol. Given a properly alkaline internal environment in the presence of good unsaturated fatty acids and B vitamins, cholesterol in the blood does not necessarily lead to artery or heart problems.

In its processing role, the liver converts simple sugar—glucose—into glycogen, which it then stores and releases when you need energy between meals. It breaks down proteins—both the ones you eat and old damaged proteins from elsewhere in your body. Then either it uses the component amino acids to make new proteins to send out to where they are needed in the body for growth and regeneration, or it discards them as toxins.

In the process of metabolizing proteins, ammonia is produced. This is a poison to humans. Normally, the liver converts this ammonia to urea and sends it to the kidneys, where it is disposed of as urine. But if there is a protein overload, the liver can neither digest it all out nor flush out all the ammonia, so it backs up into the blood, causing toxicity in the tissues.

On top of all this, the liver filters out a host of other toxins, including alcohol, drugs, chemicals, and old congested proteins. The hepatic artery carries blood right from the heart to the liver, so it is in a sense, the body's first line of defense after the intestines. If the liver gets overloaded with processing too many degraded proteins, it cannot do a good job filtering out these other toxins from the blood.

Who Should Undertake the Liver Cleanse?

Nearly everyone can benefit from the Liver Cleanse. One out of every four adult Americans has what is clinically diagnosed as a fatty liver. This can be caused by any number of factors, including obesity, drugs, alcohol, and disease. Fatty deposits make the liver sluggish, slow down metabolism, and impede proper functioning. Normally, it can take up to a year for a fatty liver to heal. By combining the One-Week Intensive Cure with the Liver Cleanse and then returning to the Maintenance Diet for Life, you can heal your liver in as little as three months. This program is also excellent for people with chronic inflammatory diseases and for those with psychiatric ailments, such as bipolar disorder, depression, and chronic fatigue.

Liver function is somewhat cyclical in nature in the sense that all the detritus it expels, including toxins and excess cholesterol, are dumped into the small intestine via the bile it produces. At the end of the digestive cycle at the bottom of the small intestine, a good deal of the bile acid is reabsorbed into the blood and transported back to the liver.

If you eat too many fatty foods and too little fiber from vegetables, fruits, and whole grains, there will be a buildup of this bile and old cholesterol in your liver and gallbladder, where it forms spongy stones. Some are tiny or pea size, but others can be quite large. Insoluble fibers from vegetables and whole grains that are not digested and remain in the intestines, bind with the fatty bile in the gut and help expel it so that it does not re-enter the cycle. This is why a diet rich in fiber lowers toxins and cholesterol and de-acidifies the body.

The Liver Cleanse works by first relieving stress on the liver. The exceedingly low-fat diet of the One-Week Intensive Cure—with no animal fat or protein at all—and the very high amount of fiber in the raw and lightly steamed vegetables bind with the bile acids and carries them out, so much less returns to the liver. The malolactic acid from the apple juice loosens the bile and helps open up the ducts. Then we give it a push with a special cocktail that forces out soft stones of old proteins, cholesterol, and toxins that have collected for years. You will be amazed at what comes out of your body.

The Liver Cleanse:
Step-by-Step Instructions

Step 1

Simply follow the One-Week Intensive Cure detailed in the previous chapter. But starting the very first day, in addition to 2 liters of water and herb tea, you must also drink 1 to 1½ liters of unsweetened apple juice or fresh cider each day.

Imported European apple juice, if you can find it, contains much less natural sugar than the typical American variety and will be easier on your system. Also, most adults find the subtler taste much more to their liking. Whichever kind you drink, it is essential that you stick with it. The apple juice ferments in your body, and the malolactic acid produced softens the bile stones and keeps the bile ducts open so they can pass. If the sugar in the juice is just too much for you, dilute it by half with water. Sip the juice slowly throughout the day in between meals.

Step 2

On Days 5, 6, and 7, when you wake up, drink a glass or two of plain warm water. Fifteen minutes later, take 2 tablespoons extra virgin olive oil blended with 2 tablespoons fresh organic lemon juice. Wait half an hour before eating breakfast.

Step 3

On the final (7th) day of the One-Week Intensive Cure, you may have breakfast and lunch, but no supper. Do not eat or drink anything except water after 2:00 P.M.

6:00 P.M. Dissolve 4 tablespoons (¼ cup) Epsom salts in 3 cups of water. Divide into 4 portions of ¾ cup each. Drink the first portion at once. Since the salts are bitter, and bitterness is detected on the back of the tongue, you may find it easier to gulp the potion down with a large straw. You may also take a few sips of water or suck on a slice of lemon to get rid of any unpleasant taste.

8:00 P.M. Drink your second ¾ cup of Epsom salts.

9:30 P.M. If you haven't had a bowel movement yet, take a water enema; this will trigger a series of bowel movements.

9:45 P.M. Squeeze enough grapefruit(s) to obtain ¾ cup strained juice—no pulp. Put the juice in a jar with ½ cup extra virgin olive oil. Cover and shake well until emulsified. Your goal is to drink this mixture at 10:00, but if you still need to visit the bathroom a few more times, you can delay it for 10 or 15 minutes. Once you take your last dose for the evening, you need to go straight to bed. Also, prepare a hot water bottle, just in case.

10:00 P.M. Stand next to your bed—don't sit. Quickly give the olive oil–grapefruit juice cocktail another shake and drink it down quickly, if possible in one go. If you cannot quaff it, you may, as before, use a large straw. You may also use a little natural brown sugar to chase it down between sips; however, the whole drink must be consumed within 5 minutes.

Immediately, lie down and do not get up for at least 20 minutes; otherwise you may not be able to release the "stones." Turn off the lights and lie on your back with your head up high. Use an extra pillow or two to keep your upper body elevated; you should sleep practically sitting up. If you experience any nausea, roll to your right side, keeping your head high, and tuck your knees in slightly toward your chest; this should provide relief. If not, press the hot water bottle gently against your liver, which is in the upper right side of your abdomen. Most people find this very soothing.

Now try to relax. Focus on your liver; and if you can, visualize the heavy mixture you have just drunk pushing the stones out of your liver and gallbladder. *You must remain perfectly still for at least 20 minutes!* This allows time for the fatty stones to move along the bile ducts and prepare to pass into the stools. You will experience no pain. All the preparations you have made and the Epsom salts will keep the bile duct valves wide open and thin the bile fluid. Go to sleep if you can.

If at any time during the night you feel the need to have a bowel movement, go to the bathroom. When you are done, check to see if there are already small gallstones, which may be green or tan colored, floating in the toilet. You may feel slightly nauseous during the night or in the early morning, but if you do, it will not last long.

Step 4

6:00–6:30 A.M. Upon awakening—but not before 6:00—drink your third ¾ cup of dissolved Epsom salts. If you are very thirsty when you wake up, you may first drink a glass of warm water before taking the salts. Rest and relax. You may feel a little low, but this will pass later on in the morning. This is a very good time to meditate. If you feel sleepy, go back to bed.

8:00–8:30 A.M. Drink your fourth and last ¾ cup of Epsom salts mixture; then simply rest. From the time you wake up until about 9:00 A.M., you may go to the bathroom many times. Most of what you evacuate will be watery, but filled with little stones. You will be surprised at how many stones you pass. Many will be the size of small peas, but there may be a few so large they will surprise you.

10:00–10:30 A.M. Slowly drink a small glass of freshly squeezed fruit juice of your choice. A half hour later, you may eat a piece of fruit. Then at noon, have a light lunch, preferably one very low in protein and fat. The one described on the first day of the Swiss Detox Diet is ideal.

Now you should feel fresh and clean. Try to stick to the Maintenance Diet for Life pretty strictly for at least 1 month. This will continue the process of purging excess proteins and toxins and seriously transition your internal environment from an acidic to an alkaline milieu. This program regulates your metabolism while it continues the purification you have jump-started. It also lightens your toxic load and boosts your immune system considerably because so many food allergens have been removed from your diet. Over time, the results of this sort of purification are truly dramatic.

CHAPTER TWELVE

Questions and Answers for Body and Soul

SOME SOLUTIONS TO THE PUZZLE

As I've mentioned many times before, Swiss biological medicine doesn't differentiate between the psychological and the physical. They are simply two different expressions of the same system. It's impossible to do something to the psyche without affecting the body and vice versa. Traditional doctors recognized this many years ago. Many of them just forgot. Let me give you an easy example.

Even when classic psychoanalysis was much more popular than it is today and talk therapy was acknowledged as being very effective at helping people in many ways, it was never very good at dealing with phobias: fear of spiders, fear of snakes, fear of heights, and the like. Getting at the psychic root of *why* a person panicked hysterically when stimulated with a specific trigger eluded psychiatrists and psychologists alike. Treatment simply was not very successful.

Then a clever researcher came up with an idea. He analyzed what happened when someone had a phobic attack and saw that, while the initial trigger as well as the fear and panic it engendered was highly emotional, the ensuing physical response of the body—the pumping of adrenaline, clenching of the muscles, racing of the pulse—reinforced those psychological symptoms. Essentially, the physical response to the psychological upset simply heightened the emotional state, amplifying the terror, which increased the physical symptoms even more. He saw that the physical and mental effects of a phobic attack consisted of a single unified cycle; they could not be separated.

Since successfully treating the phobia psychologically had eluded doctors for so long, he wondered what would happen if you broke the cycle at its physical point instead. What would happen if you taught a patient to control their attacks by soothing their body rather than their mind—relaxing their muscles, learning to breathe regularly and deeply, focusing on calming down?

It turned out that properly controlling the physical side of a phobic attack had a dramatic effect on reducing the anxiety of the phobia. His theory led to the development of Progressive Relaxation, a physical technique that proved highly effective in curing psychological phobias of all sorts.

In a similar way, the nutrition espoused by Dr. Rau's Way will over time have a dramatic effect not only on your body, but also on your psyche—on your personality and your emotions. After all, we know that they belong to one unified system. Understandably, the interaction between the health of one of your most important organs (the intestine) and its neural system (the parasympathetic unconscious nervous system) is very intense. If you eat something bad, you feel awful in a way that strongly affects your emotions and even your thinking. If you suddenly feel nauseous, your whole frame of mind turns over in a moment. Certainly, you've experienced this yourself many times—whether with a bout of food poisoning, while being seasick, or during a hangover. When drinking too much, you can go from feeling happy, carefree, and somewhat silly to being utterly miserable and wretched in just moments.

Depending upon the internal environment of your gut, within a very brief period of time, your psychological state, even the expression of your personality can change. Since this happens on such a gross level, why should the same not be true on a subtle level? So we see that even slight, permanent changes of your internal environment, such as that produced by a change in your diet, also produces changes of personality. That's one reason why people who follow Dr. Rau's Way report feeling calmer, more peaceful and relaxed, less anxious, and certainly less depressed in as little as six weeks. (It's also why the plan helps people who have been suffering with intractable mental problems like depression, attention deficit disorder, hyperactivity, and even autism.)

Practiced over time, the expression of the nutrition inside your physical body will have a marked benevolent effect on how you feel emotionally as well as physically and will alter the way you interact with the world around you. Beyond peace of mind, awareness and greater self-understanding are also cultivated.

For it's only our Western mechanical way of viewing the world that differentiates between psyche and body. In fact, the two are a single entity. Ancient medical cultures, such as the Chinese and shamanic Indian traditions, make no such separation. While Swiss biological medicine embraces the most modern diagnostic and treatment tools available, we maintain this traditional stance toward body and soul. That's one reason I ask my patients so many questions.

Dr. Rau's Questions

Like any doctor, I interview patients about why they've come to me and what is bothering them. But I find that asking people the following questions, on successive visits over a course of treatment, gives me a deeper insight into their problems from a Swiss biological medicine point of view. If you learn to ask the right questions and then learn where to find the right answers, you will uncover a lot about the cause of your problems, whether they are mildly systemic or a serious illness. And solving the puzzle of your symptoms will benefit you both physically and psychologically, which is one reason our treatment reaches such a wide range of ills.

It is my sincerest hope that by asking yourself these questions and taking time to ponder the answers, perhaps some of the pieces of the puzzle of your health and well-being will fit together. For only by understanding ourselves and our uniqueness—in body and soul—can we truly heal.

Life-Theme Questions

1. What is your main symptom and why does it bother you?

   Learning how much importance you attach to a symptom and how much it impacts your life reveals a great deal about the psychic affairs that dominate your life, about your mind-set, and about the relationship of the problem to your life. While this question gives me insight as a doctor, it is something that is important for you to ponder to help put your health in perspective.

2. Do you have any pain, and if so, where and how bad is it on a scale of one to ten?

   How you relate to a symptom and the ensuing discomfort also reveals your primal fears. Self-knowledge is always a good place to start. It can help separate out what is your real problem from peripheral disturbances.

3. What do you expect to gain from our treatments or from biological medicine, especially from the nutrition you practice at home?

   The answer to this will reveal a great deal about how much responsibility you are willing to take for your own health. Swiss biological medicine and especially Dr. Rau's Way work best when the patient makes a commitment over the long term. This answer also shows the context of the disease in your life.

Food Allergy Questions

4. Were you breast-fed as a baby, and if so, for how long?

    If you were not, the probability that you have a severe food allergy is much higher. By following Dr. Rau's Way into the Maintenance Diet for Life stage, you will learn how to identify your primary food allergies so that you can avoid them, which is essential for good health.

5. Do you have a susceptibility to infections or did you have frequent infections as a child?

    A tendency toward contracting infections indicates a blockage or overload of the immune system, which most frequently is caused by a primary food allergy. It is extremely important to identify these allergies and deal with them in order to prevent serious immune-related diseases.

6. Do you suffer from allergies or asthma or did you as a child?

    Allergy or asthma symptoms indicate a high probability that you have a food allergy or disturbance of the intestinal flora.

7. Have you had a tonsillectomy or appendectomy?

    The tonsils and appendix are both lymph organs. When they swell or get infected repeatedly, it's a sign that even your auxiliary lymph system is trying to help increase your immune reactions. Strengthening the immune system in the gut can heal tonsillitis or incipient appendicitis.

Toxic Overload Questions

8. Do you have any amalgam fillings or root canals?

   Both are the most frequent toxic loads and the most frequently overlooked causes of chronic diseases.

9. Have you taken antibiotics frequently throughout your lifetime?

   If you have, this indicates you may have a susceptibility to infections or you may have the wrong doctor.

10. Which vaccinations have you received?

    There are many chronic neurological and autoimmune diseases that are triggered as side effects of vaccinations. These are caused both by the mercury used as a preservative for the vaccine (thiomersal) and by the viruses contained in the vaccination itself, which can create the diseases themselves—for example, possibly autism from measles, multiple sclerosis (MS) from hepatitis B, and neurodermitis (children's eczema) from polio and pertussis.

Nutritional Questions

11. Do you often feel tired after meals?

    This shows poor regulation of blood sugar. A hyper-insulin reaction causes blood sugar to drop too precipitously, resulting in fatigue and grogginess for up to two hours after eating. This hyper-insulin reaction is often a cause of obesity and depression. It can also be an expression of disturbed thyroid function.

12. Do you have sudden hunger pangs so intense they often cause you to lose the ability to focus or think properly?

This indicates hypoglycemia, which is closely related to the drop in blood sugar and lack of regulation described in the answer above.

13. Are your bowel habits regular?

Chronic constipation is always an expression of either poor intestinal bacteria or a weak parasympathetic nervous system. Chronic diarrhea is nearly always related to a food allergy.

14. What foods do you not tolerate well?

Most people are not aware of their primary food allergens. Foods you know you don't tolerate well are nearly always secondary allergies or an expression of low enzymatic function. For example, if you don't digest fruit easily, chances are you are lacking the enzyme needed to process fructose, or fruit sugar.

15. How much fluid do you drink per day and what do you drink?

Drinking the wrong fluids, especially iced drinks, artificially sweetened drinks, or milk, is often the cause of diseases. Drinking copious amounts of the right fluids is essential to good health.

Some Deeper Questions

16. What scares you most . . . and why?

Fear weakens our immune system, and having hope increases the healing capacity. This question gives me an introduction into what patients may or may not really know about their disease. Sometimes misinformation, such as from Internet research or from insensitive, negative, or even fearful doctors, blocks the healing capacity. This question gives me an opportunity to give hope to the patient. Looking at your fears from a rational biological medicine point of view may well offer you the hope you need.

17. What do you feel is the cause of your disease?

This addresses the intuitive knowledge, often unconscious, that is within each and every person. It's amazing how often patients have the answer or how often they answer with uncanny self-knowledge. You may know yourself better than you're willing to acknowledge, and that insight may help you solve the puzzle of your illness.

Question for the Seriously Ill

18. Imagine a magician might come to you and fulfill one wish. Assuming that wish may not be to get healthy or to acquire magical powers to change things, what would it be?

This question can lead you into a deep understanding of what you value most in life and what change can help you heal. Even in the most serious of situations, fulfilling yourself day by day offers tremendous comfort and peace of mind and can extend both life and quality of life. Sometimes asking this question at an early stage can even save your life.

Here's what I mean. I have a good friend whom I've known for more than 30 years, but we see each other rarely. We're very different but quite close. One time when we met, he told me we had to talk. I was too busy; but he kept insisting, and finally I took the time to listen. And then he told me, "You know, Thomas, I'm your friend and I've been observing you, and I have to tell you, even though you won't want to hear it, that there is a lot you're doing wrong, and if you don't change, you're going to get sick."

He was right: I didn't want to hear what he had to say because it was unpleasant, even though deep down I knew he was right. I was lucky I had such a friend, because without his help, I wouldn't have changed. I was too stubborn and stuck in my old behavior patterns.

Sometimes a life-threatening disease can be the good friend who shows you that you have to change something—improve your diet, relieve some stress in your life, practice a regular program of exercise, spend more time with your loved ones. Whatever it is, you probably knew it already, but without the pressure of the illness, you wouldn't make the change.

Making alterations at an earlier stage, when you're not yet sick, can save your life. You can be your own best friend by paying attention, asking the right questions, and doing what your body already knows has to be done. By following this path and incorporating Dr. Rau's Way, you will solve many puzzles and perhaps surprise yourself in your potential to heal, to thrive, and even to evolve on a spiritual level.

Changing your lifestyle, especially your nutrition, will alter your attitudes and your values. It may surprise you, but in the long term, even your interests will change, and you will attain a finer level of comprehension of the natural world around you. By this I mean that changing your nutrition will mean incorporating the idea of a healthier earth in your life—physically and ethically.

The choices you make to improve your health—eating organically raised fruits and vegetables, humanely raised animals, lovingly prepared food—are incorporated into your body. As we've learned, each and every cell rebuilds periodically, and nutrition gives you the material to rebuild. So isn't it clear that when the building materials are better, the quality of the new tissues will get better. And isn't it also clear that all the energy in the nutrition is incorporated into the energy of your cells, thus connecting us intimately with the earth around us, transforming us ultimately into a better part of a better planet.

RECIPES

Snacks

Snacks are an important part of Dr. Rau's nutritional program. They help maintain a healthy blood sugar level all day and make sure you're not ravenous by mealtime. Many of these recipes could also serve as part of a composed salad plate or a light supper if accompanied by another dish.

Avocado-Cheese Melt

Baba Ghanoush

Sesame-Ginger Eggplant Spread

Sweet Potato–Pine Nut Spread

Guacamole with Baked Tortilla Chips

Lemony Hummus with Toasted Cumin Seeds

Herbed Yogurt Cheese

Pita Pizzettes with Basil Goat Cheese and Black Olive Tapenade

Spiced Steamed Chickpeas

Lemon-Rosemary White Bean Spread

White Bean and Arugula Spread with Olives and Sun-Dried Tomatoes

Avocado-Cheese Melt

You can enjoy this as a tasty snack in the middle of the afternoon; or double the portions, tuck some sprouts in the middle, and have it as a nice sandwich at lunch.

■ 1 SERVING

> 1 thin slice of spelt or whole-grain bread
>
> ½ teaspoon extra virgin olive oil
>
> ¼ ripe avocado
>
> Lemon wedge
>
> Pinch of sea salt
>
> 2 or 3 paper-thin slices of Manchego cheese

1. Toast the bread lightly. Drizzle the oil over the toast.
2. Slice the avocado as thinly as you can and arrange it over the toast. If it is too soft, cut thicker slices and mash them slightly to cover the toast. Season lightly with a squeeze of lemon juice and pinch of salt. Drape the cheese over the avocado.
3. Slip under a hot broiler for a couple of minutes, or broil in a toaster oven, just until the cheese melts. With a sharp serrated knife, cut in half or quarters.

Baba Ghanoush

Whole wheat or spelt pita triangles and Kalamata olives or carrot and zucchini sticks make great accompaniments for this Middle Eastern eggplant spread.

■ MAKES ABOUT 2 CUPS

> 2 large eggplants (about 1 pound each)
>
> ¼ cup tahini (Middle Eastern sesame seed paste)
>
> ¼ cup extra virgin olive oil

2 to 3 tablespoons fresh lemon juice

1 small garlic clove, minced

1 tablespoon chopped flat-leaf parsley

Sea salt and freshly ground black pepper

1.   Preheat the oven to 425°F. With the tip of a small knife, prick the egg-plants all over. Place on a baking sheet and roast, turning once, for 50 to 60 minutes, until the eggplants have collapsed slightly and are very soft throughout. Remove from the oven and let cool to room temperature.

2.   Cut the eggplants in half lengthwise. Scoop the eggplant pulp from the skin and drain in a sieve for about 10 minutes to remove excess liquid.

3.   Transfer the eggplant to a food processor. Add the tahini, olive oil, lemon juice, garlic, and half the parsley. Puree until smooth. Season with salt and pepper to taste. Serve with a little of the remaining chopped parsley sprinkled on top.

Sesame-Ginger Eggplant Spread

Easy to make and tempting to eat, this savory spread is good on rice crackers or as a dip for crudités.

■ MAKES ABOUT 1¾ CUPS

1 pound small Asian eggplants, skins on

4½ tablespoons extra virgin olive oil

1 tablespoon organic wheat-free tamari

1 tablespoon raw brown sugar

1 tablespoon rice vinegar

1 tablespoon finely minced fresh ginger

1 garlic clove, minced

2 teaspoons Asian sesame oil

2 tablespoons toasted sesame seeds

1. Wash and dry the eggplants. Trim off the stem ends and slice the eggplants crosswise on a diagonal into ¼-inch ovals.

2. In a wok or large skillet, heat 1½ tablespoons of the olive oil over medium-high heat. Add the eggplant and sauté, turning, until they are softened and lightly browned, 3 to 5 minutes. Repeat with the same amount of olive oil and the remaining eggplant slices. As they are done, set aside on paper towels to drain.

3. In a small bowl, combine the tamari, brown sugar, and rice vinegar; stir to dissolve the sugar. In a clean wok or large skillet, heat the remaining olive oil over medium heat. Add the ginger and garlic and stir-fry for about 30 seconds, until fragrant. Add the tamari mixture and stir briefly. Return all the fried eggplant to the pan and stir quickly to coat all the slices with sauce. Remove from the heat and transfer to a bowl. Drizzle the sesame oil over the eggplant and mash with a fork to make a coarse spread. Let cool.

4. To serve, stir half the sesame seeds into the eggplant spread. Transfer to a serving bowl and sprinkle the remaining seeds on top.

Sweet Potato–Pine Nut Spread

What we call a sweet potato is really a deep orange yam, and they are full of vitamins and minerals and low in fat. This is a healthful and satisfying spread, lovely on a simple rye cracker for a snack in between meals. It keeps well in the refrigerator for up to five days.

■ MAKES ABOUT 1 CUP

1 large sweet potato or yam (8 to 10 ounces)

2 tablespoons pine nuts (pignoli)

1 to 2 tablespoons maple syrup, to taste

1 tablespoon sunflower oil

¼ teaspoon cinnamon

Pinch of sea salt

1. Preheat the oven to 400°F. Prick the sweet potato in several places with the tip of a knife and bake for about 45 minutes, until very tender throughout. Remove from the oven and let cool slightly. Scrape the sweet potato from the skin.

2. In a small dry skillet, toast the pine nuts over medium heat, shaking the pan to stir the nuts, until they are fragrant and lightly toasted, about 3 minutes.

3. In a food processor—a mini works well here—combine the baked sweet potato and toasted pine nuts. Puree until smooth. Add 1 tablespoon of the maple syrup, the oil, cinnamon, and sea salt. Puree to blend. Taste and add up to 1 more tablespoon maple syrup if needed.

Guacamole with Baked Tortilla Chips

Avocados are one of the A-list vegetables. They are rich in potassium and healthy fats, which help maintain your blood sugar levels between meals. Guacamole is simply a Mexican word that means "avocado sauce." There are as many variations as there are cooks. Here is mine.

■ MAKES ABOUT 1¼ CUPS

> 2 ripe avocados
>
> 1 plum tomato, finely diced
>
> ¼ to ½ teaspoon grated lime or lemon zest
>
> 1½ teaspoons freshly squeezed lime or lemon juice
>
> 1 small garlic clove, minced
>
> 1 serrano chile, seeded and minced (optional)
>
> Sea salt
>
> Baked Tortilla Chips (recipe follows) or your favorite brand

1. Cut each avocado in half lengthwise. Twist the halves in opposite directions to separate. Remove and discard the pits. With an avocado

peeler or large spoon, scoop the avocado into a bowl. Mash coarsely with a fork.

2. Add the tomato, lime zest, lime juice, garlic, and chile. Mix well. Season very lightly with salt. Serve with Baked Tortilla Chips.

Baked Tortilla Chips

Allow one 6-inch tortilla for each person.

6-inch organic corn tortillas
Grape seed oil or extra virgin olive oil

1. Preheat the oven to 350°F. Brush the tortilla lightly on both sides with oil. Cut in half; then divide each half in thirds to make 6 triangles from each.

2. Spread out the tortillas chips in a single layer on a large baking sheet. Bake for about 10 minutes, until crisp.

Lemony Hummus with Toasted Cumin Seeds

Fresh lemon juice along with grated zest imparts a lovely citrus flavor to this hummus. It makes a fine snack or an excellent dip for a party. Serve with toasted whole wheat pita triangles or cut-up raw vegetables.

NOTE: The recipe halves easily. If you don't feel like toasting the seeds, simply substitute 1½ teaspoons ground cumin; you need a little more because the flavor is milder.

■ MAKES ABOUT 3 CUPS

1 teaspoon cumin seeds
2 cups cooked chickpeas, rinsed and drained

⅓ cup tahini (Middle Eastern sesame seed paste)

½ teaspoon grated lemon zest

2 to 3 tablespoons fresh lemon juice

3 tablespoons extra virgin olive oil

1 teaspoon sea salt

Paprika, sweet or hot to taste

1. In a small dry skillet, toast the cumin seeds over medium heat, shaking the pan once or twice, until they are lightly browned and fragrant, 2 to 3 minutes. Transfer to a mortar and crush lightly, or grind in a spice grinder or mini food processor.

2. Combine the chickpeas, tahini, lemon zest, 2 tablespoons of the lemon juice, olive oil, salt, and toasted cumin seeds in a food processor or blender. Add ½ cup warm water and puree until smooth.

3. Season with more lemon juice and additional salt to taste. Transfer to a bowl and serve at room temperature, with a dusting of paprika on top.

Herbed Yogurt Cheese

This is excellent as a spread, as a stuffing for raw vegetables, or to dollop as a garnish onto a soup or stew.

■ MAKES ABOUT 1 CUP

1 cup Yogurt Cheese (page 296)

1 tablespoon minced fresh chives

1 tablespoon finely chopped fresh parsley

1 tablespoon minced fresh dill or basil

Coarsely cracked black pepper

Mix together the Yogurt Cheese, chives, parsley, and dill or basil to blend well. Season with pepper to taste. Cover and refrigerate for up to 2 days before serving.

Pita Pizzettes with Basil Goat Cheese and Black Olive Tapenade

If fresh basil is not available, oregano, chives, thyme, or parsley—or a combination of any of these—would be just as appealing in this quick, nutritious snack.

■ 4 SERVINGS

> 4 ounces soft white goat cheese, at room temperature
>
> 1 tablespoon coarsely chopped fresh basil
>
> Sea salt and freshly ground pepper
>
> 4 organic sprouted wheat or whole wheat pita pockets
>
> 4 teaspoons extra virgin olive oil
>
> 8 teaspoons black olive tapenade (olive spread)

1. Preheat the oven to 375°F and set a rack in the top position. In a small bowl, blend the goat cheese with the basil. Season with salt and pepper to taste, keeping in mind that tapenade can be very salty.

2. Lay the pitas on a baking sheet and brush each one with about 1 teaspoon extra virgin olive oil. Bake for about 3 minutes to crisp slightly. Remove from the oven and let cool briefly.

3. Divide the goat cheese mixture among the 4 pitas and spread it to within ½ inch of the edges of the bread. Drop four ½-teaspoon dollops of tapenade on top of the goat cheese on each of the pitas. Swirl lightly with the back of a spoon.

4. Return to the oven and bake the pizzettes for 5 minutes, until warmed through.

Spiced Steamed Chickpeas

Star food writer Paula Wolfert tells how to steam chickpeas in her book The Slow Mediterranean Kitchen. *Soaked and then steamed without any preliminary cooking, the beans develop a delightful texture—soft but slightly chewy, great for snacking. They are best eaten hot or warm, right after cooking.*

■ MAKES ABOUT 1½ CUPS

> ½ cup dried chickpeas, rinsed and picked over
>
> 1 tablespoon extra virgin olive oil
>
> ¼ teaspoon ground cumin
>
> ¼ teaspoon Aleppo or Marash pepper or a dash of cayenne
>
> Coarse sea salt

1. Put the chickpeas in a medium bowl and add enough cold water to cover by at least 1½ inches. Let soak, changing the water several times, for at least 12 or up to 48 hours. If you soak the chickpeas longer than 12 hours, be sure to refrigerate them and don't forget to keep changing the water.
2. Steam the chickpeas over boiling water until tender, 25 to 35 minutes.
3. In a medium skillet, heat the olive oil with the cumin and pepper. When nice and hot, add the chickpeas and toss to coat them with the oil. Season with salt to taste and serve hot.

Lemon-Rosemary White Bean Spread

While this savory spread can be eaten as soon as it is made, the flavor improves if it is refrigerated for a few hours. In fact, it keeps well for up to a week, which makes it easy to keep on hand.

■ MAKES ABOUT 1¼ CUPS

> ¼ cup extra virgin olive oil
>
> 1 teaspoon minced rosemary, preferably fresh
>
> Grated zest and juice from 1 lemon
>
> ¼ teaspoon freshly ground pepper
>
> 1½ cups cooked cannellini or other white beans
>
> Sea salt

1. In a small heavy saucepan, combine the olive oil, rosemary, lemon zest, and pepper. Set over moderately low heat for about 1 minute, until the oil just begins to bubble. Remove from the heat and let steep for 10 to 15 minutes.

2. Puree the beans in a food processor. With the machine on, add the oil with the rosemary and lemon zest through the feed tube. Continue to process for at least 1 full minute, until the spread is smooth and light.

3. Blend in the lemon juice and season with salt to taste. Transfer to a covered container and refrigerate for several hours before serving.

White Bean and Arugula Spread with Olives and Sun-Dried Tomatoes

The beans must be very tender for this dish. Canned will be soft enough. If cooking them yourself, give them an extra 5 to 10 minutes. Serve the spread with raw vegetables or crackers.

■ MAKES ABOUT 2 CUPS

> 2 cups cooked or canned white beans
>
> 3 to 4 tablespoons fruity extra virgin olive oil
>
> 1 tablespoon fresh lemon juice
>
> Freshly ground pepper
>
> ⅓ cup coarsely chopped Kalamata olives
>
> ⅓ cup coarsely chopped arugula or 3 tablespoons chopped parsley
>
> ¼ cup finely diced sun-dried tomatoes (reconstituted dried or oil-packed)

1. In a large bowl, mash the beans coarsely with a fork or potato masher.
2. Add the olive oil and lemon juice and mix well to make a moist, coarse paste. Season generously with pepper.
3. Add the olives, arugula, and sun-dried tomatoes. Stir to distribute evenly.

Variation: *White Bean Bruschetta*

Make the white bean spread as directed above. Spread the mixture thickly on slabs of grilled whole grain or spelt bread that has been lightly rubbed with a cut garlic clove. Top with a drizzle of olive oil.

Soups and Chowders

Soups are an important part of Dr. Rau's nutritional program. They offer an easy and very savory way to eat more vegetables—flavorful, alkalizing, and full of vitamins and minerals. Some are a good source of essential amino acids as well. Soups and chowders also help us take in more fluids.

At the end of this section, you'll find a recipe for organic vegetable broth, in case you wish to make your own. And above all, don't forget Dr. Rau's Alkaline Soup (page 152), which should be drunk morning and evening and can be enjoyed any time of day for a pick-me-up when you are detoxifying.

Cold Avocado and Cucumber Soup
Ruby Beet Soup
Quick Broccoli Soup
Carrot-Ginger Soup
Cauliflower–Celery Root Bisque
Silky Chestnut and Parsnip Bisque with Fennel
Sweet Corn and Potato Chowder
Lentil Soup

Millet and Vegetable Soup
Minestrone
Sweet Pea Soup with Fresh Mint
Baked Potato and Fennel Soup
Roast Butternut Squash Soup
Rosemary Squash and Pear Soup
Savory White Bean Soup
Organic Vegetable Broth

Cold Avocado and Cucumber Soup

This cool, creamy summer soup requires no cooking. A swirl of goat yogurt mixed with some extra minced dill or fresh chives would make the perfect garnish.

■ 4 SERVINGS

1 large seedless cucumber or 2 large regular cucumbers

2 ripe avocados

1½ cups plain rice milk

1½ tablespoons fresh lemon juice

1 tablespoon chopped fresh dill

Sea salt and cayenne

1. Peel the cucumber, cut in half lengthwise, and scoop out any seeds with large spoon. Thickly slice the cucumber halves.
2. Halve and pit the avocados. With an avocado peeler or large spoon, scoop out the avocado.
3. Place the cucumber and avocado in a blender or food processor. Add the rice milk, lemon juice, and dill. Puree until smooth. Season with sea salt and a dash of cayenne. Transfer to a covered container and chill before serving.

Ruby Beet Soup

■ 6 SERVINGS

2 tablespoons extra virgin olive oil

¼ cup chopped leek

3 medium beets, peeled and cut into 1-inch chunks

2 medium carrots, peeled and thickly sliced

6 cups vegetable or chicken stock

Grated zest and juice from ½ orange

Grated zest and juice from ½ lemon

2 tablespoons minced fresh dill

1½ tablespoons minced fresh chives

Sea salt and freshly ground pepper

6 tablespoons plain goat yogurt

1. Heat the olive oil in a large saucepan or flameproof casserole over medium heat. Add the leek and cook until softened, 2 to 3 minutes.

2. Add the beets, carrots, and stock. Bring to a boil, reduce the heat to medium-low, cover, and cook for 25 to 30 minutes, until the beets are tender. Remove the saucepan from the heat, uncover, and let cool for 15 minutes.

3. In a blender or food processor, puree the soup in batches until smooth. Do not overfill, because this will be messy if it flies out.

4. Return the pureed soup to the saucepan. Add the grated orange and lemon zest and half the dill and chives. Season with salt and pepper to taste. Simmer for 5 minutes. Stir in the orange and lemon juice and serve hot or cold, with a dollop of yogurt and the remaining herbs sprinkled on top.

Quick Broccoli Soup

If you have water saved from steaming vegetables, this is a very good place to use it. Otherwise, any organic vegetable broth or even chicken stock will do. Broccoli stems are easily peeled by slipping the edge of a small knife under the skin and pulling back, as you would do to string celery, for instance. The peel will come right off.

NOTE: If you are avoiding gluten, omit the flour and instead cook 1 small baking potato, peeled and diced, with the broccoli.

■ 6 SERVINGS

> 1 head of broccoli (1¼ to 1½ pounds)
>
> 3 tablespoons extra virgin olive oil or unsalted butter
>
> ¼ cup thinly sliced leek
>
> 2 tablespoons spelt flour
>
> 5 cups vegetable steaming water or organic broth
>
> ¼ teaspoon freshly grated nutmeg
>
> 3 to 4 tablespoons heavy cream
>
> Sea salt and freshly ground pepper

1. Trim off the bottom of the broccoli stems. Cut the florets off the stems and divide them into small pieces. Peel the stems and cut into ½-inch pieces.

2. In a large saucepan or flameproof casserole, heat the oil or melt the butter over medium heat. Add the leek, cover, and cook for 3 minutes. Uncover, add the flour, and cook, stirring, for 1 to 2 minutes without allowing it to color.

3. Whisk in 1 cup of the vegetable water or broth and bring to a boil, whisking until the liquid is smooth and thickened. Whisk in the rest of the broth. Add the broccoli stems and nutmeg and bring to a boil. Reduce the heat slightly and cook, partially covered, for 10 minutes.

4. Add the broccoli florets and cook for 3 minutes. Add the cream and

remove from the heat. Puree right in the pot with an immersion stick blender or in batches as necessary in a blender or food processor. Season with salt and pepper to taste. Reheat, if necessary, before serving.

Carrot-Ginger Soup

A subtle hint of curry seasoning enlivened with fresh ginger makes this pretty orange soup a fine way to start a meal. It keeps well for up to three days.

■ 4 TO 6 SERVINGS

2 tablespoons extra virgin olive oil

¼ cup thinly sliced white of leek

2 teaspoons minced fresh ginger

5 medium carrots, peeled and sliced

1½ teaspoons Madras curry powder or 1 teaspoon ground cumin

6 cups vegetable or chicken broth

Sea salt

1. Heat the olive oil in a large saucepan or flameproof casserole over medium-low heat. Add the leek and ginger, cover, and cook for 3 minutes. Add the carrots and curry powder, raise the heat to medium-high, and cook, stirring often, for 2 minutes.
2. Add the broth and bring to a boil. Reduce the heat to low, cover, and simmer for 20 minutes, or until the carrots are very tender. Remove from the heat, uncover, and let the soup cool for 15 minutes.
3. Puree the soup in the pot with an immersion stick blender or in batches in a blender or food processor. Reheat the soup and season with salt to taste before serving.

Cauliflower–Celery Root Bisque

Celery root, which is sometimes called celeriac, is a very alkalizing root vegetable that's excellent both grated raw and cooked. If you have trouble finding it in your market, this soup is also delicious made with the cauliflower alone. If you omit the celery root, add ¾ teaspoon paprika, preferably smoked Spanish paprika, when you add the cauliflower.

■ 4 TO 6 SERVINGS

> 3 tablespoons extra virgin olive oil
>
> ¼ cup minced leek (white and pale green)
>
> 1 large celery root, peeled and cut into ¾-inch pieces
>
> 6 cups vegetable or chicken broth
>
> 1 head of cauliflower, trimmed into florets
>
> 3 tablespoons heavy cream
>
> Sea salt and freshly grated nutmeg
>
> Dash of cayenne

1. In a large saucepan or flameproof casserole, heat the olive oil over medium heat. Add the leek and cook, stirring, until softened, 3 to 5 minutes.

2. Add the celery root and stir to coat with the oil. Pour in the broth and bring to a boil. Reduce the heat and simmer, partially covered, for 10 minutes.

3. Add the cauliflower and continue to cook for 10 to 15 minutes longer, or until all the vegetables are soft.

4. Add the cream to the soup. Puree in the pot with an immersion stick blender or in batches in a blender or food processor. Season with salt, nutmeg, and cayenne to taste.

Silky Chestnut and Parsnip Bisque with Fennel

Fennel and chestnuts complement each other beautifully. This is a delicious soup, fine enough for company.

▧ 4 TO 6 SERVINGS

2 tablespoons extra virgin olive oil

3 tablespoons thinly sliced leek (white and pale green)

1 teaspoon fennel seeds, lightly crushed

1 small fennel bulb, coarsely chopped

2 medium-large parsnips, peeled and diced

1 cup cooked, peeled chestnuts

6 cups vegetable or chicken broth

3 tablespoons heavy cream

Coarse sea salt and freshly ground pepper

1. Heat the olive oil in a large saucepan or flameproof casserole over medium heat. Add the leek, fennel seeds, and chopped fresh fennel. Cook, stirring occasionally, until the leek and fennel are slightly softened, about 3 minutes.

2. Add the parsnips and chestnuts. Pour in the broth and bring to a boil. Reduce the heat and simmer, partially covered, until the parsnips are soft, about 20 minutes.

3. Add the cream. Puree the soup until smooth in the pot with an immersion blender or in batches in a blender or food processor. Before serving, reheat the bisque over medium-low heat and season with salt and pepper to taste.

Sweet Corn and Potato Chowder

Corn is not as seasonal as it used to be, but the best is still fresh and local. Serve this rich, chunky chowder with a sprinkling of minced chives or parsley for added color.

NOTE: If for any reason, the chowder is not as thick as you like it, dissolve 1 to 2 teaspoons cornstarch in ¼ cup cold water and stir into the boiling soup. It will thicken within 1 or 2 minutes.

■ 6 SERVINGS

> 3 ears of fresh corn
> 3 tablespoons unsalted butter
> 3 tablespoons minced white of leek
> 2 medium-large Yukon gold potatoes (¾ to 1 pound), peeled and cut into
>   ½-inch dice
> 1 teaspoon savory or thyme leaves
> 2 cups vegetable or chicken broth
> Sea salt and freshly ground pepper

1. In a large saucepan, bring 6 cups of nonchlorinated water to a boil. Add the corn and cook until just tender, about 3 minutes. Remove the corn, reserving the water in the pan.

2. As soon as the corn is cool enough to handle, use a large, sharp knife to cut the kernels from the cobs. Run the back of the knife down the cobs, pressing firmly, to squeeze out the rest of the corn "cream." Return the cobs to the water and boil for 10 to 15 minutes. Strain, reserving the corn stock.

3. In a clean large saucepan or flameproof casserole, melt the butter over medium heat. Add the leek and cook until softened, about 3 minutes.

4. Add the potatoes and savory and pour in the broth and corn stock. Bring to a boil, reduce the heat, and cook until the potatoes are ten-

der, 10 to 15 minutes. Add the corn kernels and "cream" and cook for 2 to 3 minutes longer.

5. Scoop out 1½ cups of the soup and puree in a blender or food processor. Return to the pot. Simmer for 5 minutes. Season with salt and pepper to taste. Serve hot.

Lentil Soup

Lentil soup has a way of growing. If you put it away and reheat it, it will have thickened and will need to be thinned with a little more water or stock. You will end up with more soup, which may need a little extra seasoning but will still be full of flavor. This is a highly nutritious soup that is ideal for supper, especially during the chillier months.

■ 6 TO 8 SERVINGS

3 tablespoons extra virgin olive oil

2 celery ribs, finely diced

2 medium carrots, peeled and finely diced

2 medium white turnips, peeled and finely diced

1 cup lentils

6 cups vegetable or chicken broth

1 dried chipotle chile

1 teaspoon thyme leaves, preferably fresh

1 whole clove, crushed

2 to 3 teaspoons cider vinegar

Sea salt and freshly ground pepper

1. Heat the olive oil in a large saucepan or flameproof casserole over medium heat. Add the celery, carrots, and turnips and stir to coat with the oil. Cover and cook for 3 to 5 minutes to soften slightly.

2. Add the lentils and stir to mix them with the oil and vegetables. Add the broth, chile, thyme, clove, and 2 cups of water. Bring to a boil, re-

duce the heat, and simmer, partially covered, for 10 minutes. Remove and discard the chile. (If you want the soup spicier, leave it in for another 5 to 10 minutes.)

3. Continue to cook the soup until the lentils are tender, 25 to 35 minutes longer. Stir in the vinegar and season with salt and pepper to taste.

Millet and Vegetable Soup

This is a recipe from Irene Guler of the Hotel Säntis in Switzerland, which houses many of the patients from the Paracelsus Clinic. Irene makes sure everyone has exactly the diet they are prescribed. This simple soup is good for just about everyone. To save effort, she cuts the carrots and celery root into large chunks and dices them finely after they are cooked.

■ 4 SERVINGS

1 cup millet

2 tablespoons extra virgin olive oil

2 medium carrots, peeled and halved

1 small celery root, peeled and cut into large chunks

2 teaspoons vegetable bouillon powder

1 tablespoon chopped fresh chervil, lovage, or parsley

1. In a large saucepan, toast the millet in the olive oil over medium heat, stirring often, until the millet is fragrant but not browned, about 3 minutes.

2. Pour in 6 cups of nonchlorinated water. Add the carrots, celery root, and vegetable bouillon. Bring to a boil, reduce the heat to medium-low, and cook until the vegetables and millet are soft, 20 to 25 minutes.

3. With a large slotted spoon, transfer the vegetable pieces to a cutting board. Let them cool, then cut into fine dice and return to the soup. Reheat before serving and garnish with coarsely chopped chervil.

Minestrone

Here's a lovely light version of the classic Italian garden vegetable soup. It's particularly nice in late summer or early fall, when all the vegetables are locally available. To turn it into a more substantial dish, you can add a cup of cooked cannellini beans and/or 1 cup ditallini or elbow pasta cooked just until al dente.

■ 6 SERVINGS

3 tablespoons extra virgin olive oil, plus more for serving

1 small leek (white and tender green), chopped

1 large carrot, peeled and diced

1 large celery rib, diced

1 tablespoon tomato paste

1 teaspoon dried oregano

Sea salt and freshly ground pepper

2 medium organic red potatoes, scrubbed and diced

4 ounces green beans, trimmed and cut into ¾-inch lengths (about 1 cup)

1 medium zucchini, trimmed and diced

3 tablespoons chopped fresh basil

Grated Pecorino Romano cheese

1. Heat the olive oil in a large soup pot or flameproof casserole over medium heat. Add the leek, carrot, and celery. Cover and cook until the leek is softened, about 3 minutes. Add the tomato paste and oregano and cook for 2 minutes longer.

2. Pour in 8 cups of nonchlorinated water and bring to a boil, stirring to dissolve the tomato paste. Season with 1 teaspoon salt and ¼ teaspoon pepper. Add the potatoes, reduce the heat to medium-low, and cook, partially covered, for 10 minutes.

3. Add the green beans and cook for 5 minutes. Add the zucchini and half the basil and cook for 5 minutes longer or until zucchini is just tender. Season with additional salt and pepper to taste.

4. To serve, ladle into bowls and sprinkle the remaining basil on top. Pass a bowl of grated Romano cheese and a cruet of olive oil to drizzle on top.

Sweet Pea Soup with Fresh Mint

Of course, this soup would be amazing with fresh peas from your garden or your local farmer's market. But you'd have to have a lot of help shelling them. Peas are one vegetable that freezes well. Besides saving a great deal of effort, frozen lets you enjoy this delightful, subtle soup all year round.

■ 6 SERVINGS

2 tablespoons extra virgin olive oil

2 tablespoons minced leek (white part only)

2 celery ribs, chopped

6 cups vegetable or chicken broth

2 pounds frozen baby peas, thawed

¼ cup heavy cream (optional)

⅓ cup lightly packed fresh mint leaves

Sea salt and freshly ground pepper

1. Heat the oil in a large saucepan or flameproof casserole over medium heat. Add the leek and celery and cook until slightly softened, about 3 minutes.

2. Add the broth and peas and bring to a boil. Immediately remove from the heat so the peas don't overcook. Pour in the cream and add the mint. Let the soup stand until cooled slightly.

3. Puree the soup in the pot with an immersion stick blender or in batches in a blender or food processor. Season with salt and pepper to taste. Reheat gently and strain through a mesh sieve, if desired, for an absolutely smooth texture before serving.

Baked Potato and Fennel Soup

Baking the vegetables first, instead of sautéeing them, intensifies their flavor as well as bringing out their natural sweetness.

■ 6 SERVINGS

2 medium-large Yukon gold potatoes, peeled and quartered

2 medium-large fennel bulbs, trimmed and thickly sliced

1 small leek (white and tender green), thinly sliced

3 tablespoons extra virgin olive oil

Coarse sea salt and freshly ground pepper

6 cups vegetable or chicken broth

1. Preheat the oven to 375°F. In a large baking dish, toss the potatoes, fennel, and leek with 2 tablespoons of olive oil. Season lightly with salt and pepper. Roast the vegetables for 30 minutes, or until they are tender and the fennel is lightly colored.

2. In batches in a blender or food processor, puree the roasted vegetables with the broth until smooth. As each batch is pureed, pour it into a large saucepan.

3. Bring the soup to a boil, reduce the heat, and simmer for 5 minutes. Season with additional salt and pepper to taste. Ladle into bowls and drizzle ½ teaspoon olive oil on top of each serving.

Roast Butternut Squash Soup

All the winter squashes are nutritious: high in fiber and vitamin A, they also contain vitamin C, magnesium, manganese, and potassium. But few exhibit as fine an intensity of flavor as butternut squash. If you have a hand-held stick blender, you can whip up this soup in a flash in a single pot. Toasted squash or pumpkin seeds and a drizzle of pumpkin seed oil make a nice garnish. This soup freezes perfectly.

■ 6 SERVINGS

> 1 butternut squash (1½ to 2 pounds)
>
> 3 tablespoons extra virgin olive oil
>
> 1 tablespoon chopped fresh ginger
>
> ¼ teaspoon ground allspice
>
> 6 cups vegetable or chicken broth
>
> 1 bay leaf
>
> Sea salt and freshly ground pepper

1. Preheat the oven to 350°F. Split the squash lengthwise in half and scoop out the seeds. Place cut-side down on an oiled baking sheet.
2. Bake the squash for 45 minutes, or until tender. As soon as it is cool enough to handle, scoop the flesh from the skin and reserve.
3. Heat the olive oil in a large saucepan over medium-low heat. Add the ginger and allspice and cook for 2 minutes. Add the squash, broth, bay leaf, and 1 cup of nonchlorinated water. Bring to a boil, reduce the heat, and simmer, partially covered, for 20 minutes.
4. Remove and discard the bay leaf. Puree the soup in the pot with an immersion blender; or transfer in batches to a blender or food processor and puree until smooth. Reheat if necessary. Season with salt and pepper to taste before serving.

Rosemary Squash and Pear Soup

No one will be able to identify the pear, but it contributes a lovely natural sweetness and breadth of flavor to this sumptuous soup. Enrich, if you like, with a small swirl of plain goat yogurt.

■ 6 SERVINGS

½ buttercup squash (2 pounds)

3 tablespoons extra virgin olive oil

1 medium leek (white and pale green), chopped

2 Anjou or Bosc pears, peeled, cored, and cut into chunks

2 teaspoons minced fresh rosemary, plus small sprigs for garnish

½ teaspoon freshly grated nutmeg

½ teaspoon coarse sea salt

Dash of cayenne

4 cups chicken broth

¼ cup heavy cream or soy creamer

2 teaspoons honey

1. Preheat the oven to 375°F. Roast the squash cut-side down until just tender, 35 to 40 minutes. When cool enough to handle, scoop out and discard any seeds and membranes. Remove the skin and cut the squash into large chunks.

2. In a large flameproof casserole or soup pot, heat the olive oil over medium heat. Add the leek and cook until softened, about 3 minutes. Add the pears and season them with the minced rosemary, nutmeg, sea salt, and a dash of cayenne. Add the squash and pour in enough broth to cover. If necessary, add additional stock or water.

3. Bring to a boil, reduce the heat, and simmer, partially covered, until the pears are soft, about 20 minutes. Add the cream and honey. Puree the soup until smooth in the pot with an immersion stick blender or in batches in a blender or food processor.

4. Reheat and season with additional salt and cayenne to taste. Serve garnished with a small sprig of rosemary.

Savory White Bean Soup

What better supper for a cold wintry day than a bowl of hot bean soup. Begin with a small salad and serve some nice crusty bread with goat or sheep cheese on the side.

■ 6 SERVINGS

> 3 tablespoons extra virgin olive oil, plus more for serving
>
> 2 medium carrots, peeled and finely diced
>
> 2 medium celery ribs, finely diced
>
> 1 garlic clove, minced
>
> 2 teaspoons finely chopped fresh winter savory or thyme leaves
>
> 2 cups cooked or canned white beans
>
> 6 cups vegetable broth
>
> 1 tablespoon wine vinegar or rice vinegar
>
> Sea salt and freshly ground pepper

1. Heat the olive oil in a large soup pot or flameproof casserole over medium heat. Add the carrots, celery, garlic, and savory and cook, stirring occasionally, until the celery softens, 3 to 5 minutes.
2. Add the beans and stir to mix with the vegetables. Pour in the broth and bring to a boil. Reduce the heat to low, partially cover, and simmer for 20 minutes.
3. Scoop out 2 to 3 cups of soup with beans and puree in a blender or food processor. Return the puree to the pot. Simmer for 5 minutes longer.
4. Add the vinegar and season the soup with salt and pepper to taste. Serve hot. Pass a cruet of extra virgin olive oil at the table.

Organic Vegetable Broth

There are several ways to obtain the vegetable broth you need for many of the recipes in this book: You can buy it easily not only in health-food stores, but in the natural foods section of many supermarkets. You can save up all the water from steaming vegetables throughout the week. You can "cheat" and mix up some instant stock by combining a good brand of powdered vegetable bouillon with boiling water; just watch the sodium content of these powders. Or if you feel enterprising, you can make up a batch of broth from fresh organic vegetables as directed below.

■ MAKES 8 CUPS

2 large celery ribs, chopped

1 large zucchini, sliced

1 large carrot, peeled and chopped

1 leek with 1 inch green top, washed well, trimmed and chopped

1 celery root, peeled and chopped

1 bay leaf

6 large sprigs Italian parsley

6 sprigs fresh thyme

1 teaspoon whole black peppercorns

Coarse sea salt

1. Combine all the ingredients except the salt in a large saucepan or small stockpot. Add 8 cups of nonchlorinated water. Bring to a boil, reduce the heat, and simmer for 1 hour. If the liquid reduces too much, add more water.

2. Strain into a bowl, then ladle into plastic containers and refrigerate or freeze until needed. This stock will keep well in the refrigerator for up to 4 days and in the freezer for up to 2 months.

The Salad Bar

Once you begin to see the delicious possibilities of mixing and matching vegetables for beautiful, simple composed salads, I'm convinced this will become one of your favorite parts of eating Dr. Rau's Way. Since the goal is to work your way up to eating half your calorie intake from raw vegetables, nuts, grains and seeds, a large main-course salad at lunch is a great way to go. Some of my favorite salads are included here along with a few side salads and even a salsa.

Arugula Salad with Glazed Figs and Goat Cheese
Avocado Salad with Strawberry Sauce
Avocado, Corn, and Black Bean Salsa
Celery Rémoulade
Crunchy Salad with Sunflower Seeds and Zesty Sprouts
    Sesame Ginger Vinaigrette
Shredded Beet and Carrot Salad
Marinated Roasted Beets
Asian Sesame Slaw
Corn, Rice, and Pea Salad

Green Beans with Thai-Style Sesame Sauce

Fava Bean and Artichoke Salad

Chopped Greek Salad with Cauliflower, Olives, and Feta Cheese

Swiss Potato Salad

Quinoa Salad

    Sweet-Tart Salad Dressing

Baby Spinach Salad with Carrots, Beets, and Roquefort Cheese

Arugula Salad with Glazed Figs and Goat Cheese

When fresh figs and arugula are in season, this lovely salad can serve as either a starter or as a light main course. Many people love the peppery bite of fresh arugula. If it is too strong for you, mix it with an equal amount of baby field greens (mesclun). Serve with toasted whole-grain bread brushed with olive oil.

▓ 4 SERVINGS

> 4 cups loosely packed arugula, tough stems removed
>
> 1½ tablespoons extra virgin olive oil
>
> 1 tablespoon balsamic vinegar
>
> 4 Glazed Figs with Chestnut Honey and Cashews (page 291)
>
> 2 ounces mild white goat cheese, cut into 4 rounds, at room temperature
>
> 1 lime
>
> Coarsely cracked black pepper

1. Toss the arugula with the olive oil and vinegar. Divide among 4 plates.
2. Arrange a glazed fig on each plate along with a round of goat cheese.
3. Squeeze the lime juice over the figs and garnish each salad with a light sprinkling of coarsely cracked pepper.

Avocado Salad with Strawberry Sauce

Pink and green, this pretty salad can take its place at the finest of dinner parties or delight your family any day of the week. Be sure the avocados are the creamy Hass variety.

▓ 4 SERVINGS

> 1 small bunch of arugula

12 strawberries

2 tablespoons sunflower oil

1 tablespoon balsamic vinegar

2 teaspoons fresh lemon juice

2 avocados

1. Rinse and dry the arugula. Trim off any tough stems at the bottom. Make 4 small bouquets of the arugula and place to one side of each of 4 plates.

2. In a blender or mini food processor, combine 8 of the strawberries with the sunflower oil, balsamic vinegar, and lemon juice. Puree until the strawberry dressing is smooth.

3. Cut each avocado in half and remove the pits. With a large spoon or avocado peeler, scoop out each avocado half in one piece. Cut the avocado halves lengthwise into slices and fan out on the plates. Drizzle about 1 tablespoon of the dressing over each avocado half and garnish each plate with 1 of the remaining strawberries, halved or sliced. Pass the remaining dressing.

Avocado, Corn, and Black Bean Salsa

A colorful addition to a composed salad plate, this piquant salsa can also be served with grilled chicken, fish, or veggie burgers.

■ MAKES ABOUT 1½ CUPS

1 teaspoon cumin seeds

1 large ripe but firm avocado

Juice of 1 lime

½ cup cooked or canned black beans

½ cup corn kernels—fresh, canned, or thawed frozen

⅓ cup finely diced red bell pepper

1 tablespoon sunflower oil

2 teaspoons chopped fresh oregano or parsley

1 pickled jalapeño pepper, minced (optional)

1. In a small skillet, toast the cumin seeds over medium heat until fragrant and lightly browned, 2 to 3 minutes. Let cool slightly, then crush coarsely.
2. Split the avocado in half and remove the pit. With a large spoon, scoop out the avocado and finely dice.
3. In a medium bowl, toss the avocado with the lime juice to prevent discoloration. Add the toasted cumin seeds, beans, corn, bell pepper, sunflower oil, oregano, and jalapeño pepper. Toss lightly to mix.

Celery Rémoulade

It's surprising how a recipe so simple can be so flavorful. In France, this dish is often served by itself as first course, and you certainly can do that, but it's also very nice as one element of a composed salad. Celery root will darken if left to stand, so be sure to toss it with the dressing as soon as you shred it. The lemon juice will keep it white.
■ 4 TO 6 SERVINGS

1 small celery root (celeriac)

¼ cup extra virgin olive oil

3 tablespoons fresh lemon juice

1 teaspoon Dijon mustard

Sea salt and freshly ground pepper

1. With a large sharp knife, cut away the tough outer skin of the celery root. Cut the vegetable into pieces that will fit in the tube of your food processor and shred with the grating disk.
2. In a mixing bowl, whisk together the olive oil, lemon juice, and mustard. Add the shredded celery root and toss to mix well. Season with salt and pepper to taste; you won't need much.

Crunchy Salad with Sunflower Seeds and Zesty Sprouts

Color and texture are important for food to be satisfying, especially when you have previously been eating a lot of meat.

■ 4 SERVINGS

8 large radishes, thinly sliced

2 medium carrots, peeled and thinly sliced

1 medium green bell pepper or ½ green and ½ red, cut into very thin
slices

2 cups lightly packed zesty sprouts, such as radish and alfalfa sprouts
(about 2 ounces)

⅓ cup Sesame-Ginger Vinaigrette (recipe follows)

¼ cup sunflower seeds

1 tablespoon sesame seeds

1. In a salad bowl, combine the radishes, carrots, and bell pepper. Shake
    the sprouts over the salad to distribute them evenly. Drizzle on the
    dressing and toss to mix. Let stand for 5 to 10 minutes to allow the
    dressing to permeate the radishes.

2. Add the sunflower seeds and toss to mix. Divide the salad among 4
    plates. Sprinkle the sesame seeds on top.

Sesame-Ginger Vinaigrette

Make up a batch of this enticing dressing for whenever you need it. Store in the refrigerator in a tightly closed glass jar for up to a week.

■ MAKES ABOUT 1 CUP

½ cup extra virgin olive oil

¼ cup rice vinegar

3 tablespoons Asian sesame oil

1 teaspoon organic wheat-free tamari

1 teaspoon minced fresh ginger

Put all the ingredients in a jar, close the lid tightly, and shake.

Shredded Beet and Carrot Salad

Because the natural sugars in these vegetables are tightly bound in their tough fibers, the slow release into your bloodstream will keep your energy level on an even keel for hours. This pretty salad keeps well in the refrigerator for up to four days.

■ 4 TO 6 SERVINGS

2 medium-small beets

2 large carrots

1½ tablespoons balsamic vinegar

1½ tablespoons sunflower oil

1. Peel the raw beets and carrots. Using the shredding disk of a food processor or the large holes of a hand grater, shred the vegetables.
2. Toss the shredded beets and carrots with the balsamic vinegar and sunflower oil. Serve at once or cover and refrigerate for up to 3 days.

Marinated Roasted Beets

Beets are a wonderful cleansing vegetable. Keep a batch of these on hand to sprinkle over salads for both color and flavor.

■ MAKES ABOUT 1½ CUPS

1 pound fresh beets

2 tablespoons balsamic or sherry vinegar

2 teaspoons sunflower oil

1. Preheat the oven to 400°F. Rinse the beets well and wrap them in a double thickness of aluminum foil. Roast for 45 to 60 minutes, depending on the size, until the beets are just tender.
2. Let the beets cool, then trim the tops and bottoms and rub off the skin. Cut the beets into whatever size dice you like or into slices.
3. Toss the beets with the vinegar and sunflower oil. Let stand at room temperature for at least 1 hour before using, or cover and refrigerate for up to 5 days.

Asian Sesame Slaw

This delightful slaw changes character over time. Freshly made, it's bright and crisp. By the third day, it will have softened and absorbed more of the dressing.

■ 4 TO 6 SERVINGS

¼ medium-large green cabbage

2 tablespoons rice vinegar

1 tablespoon fresh lemon juice

1 tablespoon Asian sesame oil

½ teaspoon coarse sea salt

1 tablespoon sesame seeds

1. Either thinly slice the cabbage with a large knife or shred in a food processor. There should be about 6 cups.

2. In a medium bowl, combine the shredded cabbage with the rice vinegar, lemon juice, sesame oil, salt, and half the sesame seeds. Toss to mix well.

3. Eat at once while crisp, or cover and refrigerate for up to 3 days. Garnish with the remaining sesame seeds just before eating.

Corn, Rice, and Pea Salad

Here's a protein-rich salad high in essential amino acids. Serve as a side dish or as part of a composed salad plate.

■ 4 TO 6 SERVINGS

1 cup basmati or jasmine rice

2 tablespoons rice vinegar

1 tablespoon fresh lime juice

2 tablespoons sunflower oil

Sea salt and freshly ground pepper

1½ cups corn kernels—cooked fresh, thawed frozen, or vacuum packed

1 cup frozen baby peas, thawed

1½ tablespoons minced fresh chives

1. Cook the rice in 1¾ cups of lightly salted water until tender, about 15 minutes. Transfer to a bowl and let cool.

2. Toss the warm rice with the vinegar, lime juice, and sunflower oil. Season with salt and pepper to taste. Add the corn, peas, and chives and toss lightly to mix. Serve at room temperature.

Green Beans with Thai-Style Sesame Sauce

A play on green beans in peanut sauce, this is a tantalizing salad your whole family will love. If you have no digestive problems, enliven to taste with crushed hot red pepper.

■ 3 OR 4 SERVINGS

½ pound green beans, preferably small, cut into 1-inch lengths

2 tablespoons natural cashew butter

1 tablespoon Asian sesame oil

1 tablespoon rice vinegar

2 teaspoons honey

1½ teaspoons organic wheat-free tamari

1 teaspoon grated fresh ginger

1. Steam the green beans over boiling water until just tender.
2. In a medium bowl, blend together the cashew butter, sesame oil, vinegar, honey, tamari, and ginger. Add the beans and toss to coat. Serve at room temperature.

Fava Bean and Artichoke Salad

Direct from the Italian countryside. This delightful salad makes a lovely first course or an excellent addition to any composed salad plate. The recipe will serve four people as a luncheon salad, six as a side dish.

■ 4 TO 6 SERVINGS

2 globe artichokes

3 tablespoons fresh lemon juice

2 cups shelled fava beans, from about 2 pounds fresh (or use thawed frozen)

¼ cup extra virgin olive oil

2 tablespoons coarsely chopped fresh mint or parsley

1 small garlic clove, minced

½ cup sun-dried tomato strips (reconstituted dried or oil packed)

Sea salt and freshly ground pepper

2 ounces aged Manchego cheese, in one piece

1. Trim the artichokes down to their hearts. Cook in a medium saucepan of boiling salted water with 1 tablespoon of the lemon juice until they are just tender but still quite firm, 10 to 12 minutes. It's better to undercook the artichokes rather than overcook them. Drain and rinse under cold running water. As soon as the artichokes are cool enough to handle, scoop out the hairy chokes. Thinly slice the artichoke hearts.

2. Cook the shelled fava beans in boiling water for 2 to 3 minutes, depending upon size. Immediately drain and rinse under cold running water. Drain again, then peel the beans. Do this by pinching off a small piece of skin and gently squeezing the bean out.

3. In a medium bowl, mix the olive oil, remaining 2 tablespoons lemon juice, mint, and garlic. Add the sliced artichokes, fava beans, and sun-dried tomatoes. Toss lightly to coat with the dressing. Season with salt and pepper to taste.

4. To serve, mound the salad on individual plates and with a cheese knife or swivel-bladed vegetable peeler, shave paper-thin slices of the cheese on top.

Chopped Greek Salad with Cauliflower, Olives, and Feta Cheese

Chopping all the vegetables not only makes this tempting salad easy to eat, it makes the vitamins and minerals more accessible. Still, be sure to chew all raw vegetables very well. Don't skimp on the olive oil here. Remember, it's the oil combined with the cellulose fiber that's so good for your gut.

■ 4 SERVINGS

1 head of romaine lettuce

1 cup cauliflower florets

1 garlic clove, minced

1 teaspoon dried oregano

Coarse sea salt and freshly ground pepper

3 tablespoons fresh lemon juice

⅓ cup extra virgin olive oil

12 grape tomatoes, halved

2 carrots, peeled and diced

½ green bell pepper, diced

12 Kalamata, Gaeta, or other black olives

2 ounces feta cheese, finely diced

1. Separate the romaine leaves and cut off the very bottoms. Cut the leaves lengthwise in half right through the whitish rib, then cut crosswise into ribbons.

2. Steam the cauliflower over boiling water for 2 minutes, just to soften slightly. Or you can use the florets raw. Chop into ½-inch pieces.

3. In a salad bowl, mash the garlic with the oregano and coarse salt and pepper to taste. Stir in the lemon juice and olive oil. Add the cauliflower and tomato halves to the dressing and toss to coat. Let marinate for 2 minutes.

4. Add the carrots, bell pepper, and lettuce. Toss to coat. Serve the salad with the olives and feta cheese sprinkled on top.

Swiss Potato Salad

In this country, we're not used to adding raw leek to food, but the pale green part, finely chopped and used in small amounts, makes a fine substitute for onion, which is not allowed on Dr. Rau's diet.

▓ 4 SERVINGS

> 3 medium Yukon gold potatoes (about 1 pound)
> 2 tablespoons finely chopped pale green of leek
> 3 tablespoons extra virgin olive oil
> 1½ tablespoons fresh lemon juice
> Sea salt and freshly ground pepper

1. Put the potatoes in a saucepan, cover with lightly salted water, and bring to a boil. Cook until the potatoes are tender to the center when pierced with the tip of a small knife, 15 to 20 minutes. Drain and rinse under cold running water until cool enough to handle.
2. Peel off the skins and cut the potatoes into slices or chunks. Add the leeks and toss while still warm with the olive oil and lemon juice. Season with salt and pepper to taste.

Quinoa Salad

This is one of the salads Irene Guler often serves at the Culinarium, the luncheon restaurant attached to the Paracelsus Clinic. There is always an enticing assortment of greens, shredded vegetables, seeds, and a grain salad like this one, so guests can compose their own salad plates.

▓ 4 SERVINGS

> 1 cup quinoa
> 2 carrots, peeled and shredded
> ½ cup finely diced red bell pepper

½ cup finely diced yellow bell pepper

½ cup currants

2 tablespoons chopped fresh parsley

1 tablespoon minced fresh chives

Sweet-Tart Salad Dressing (recipe follows)

1. Rinse the quinoa in a bowl of water several times, rubbing it lightly between your hands. Drain well. In a small saucepan, bring 4 cups of lightly salted water to a boil. Add the quinoa, reduce the heat to low, cover, and cook for 10 minutes. Remove from the heat and let stand, covered, for 10 to 15 minutes. Turn the quinoa out into a bowl and fluff. Cover and refrigerate until chilled. (The quinoa can be cooked a day ahead.)

2. Put the quinoa in a large serving bowl. Add the carrots, red and yellow bell peppers, currants, parsley, and chives; toss lightly to mix. Drizzle on the dressing and toss to coat evenly. Serve at room temperature or slightly chilled.

Sweet-Tart Salad Dressing

■ MAKES ABOUT ½ CUP

¼ cup extra virgin olive oil

3 tablespoons balsamic vinegar

2 tablespoons pear nectar or 2 teaspoons honey

1 teaspoon vegetable bouillon powder

Sea salt and freshly ground pepper

In a small bowl, whisk together the olive oil, balsamic vinegar, pear nectar, and bouillon powder. Season with salt and pepper to taste.

Baby Spinach Salad with Carrots, Beets, and Roquefort Cheese

Baby spinach is so easy to use today because there are excellent organic brands that come ready to use. This salad is both beautiful and delicious enough to serve as a starter for company.

■ 4 SERVINGS

2 medium carrots

1 medium or 2 small beets

1 package (12 ounces) baby spinach

3 tablespoons extra virgin olive oil

1½ tablespoons sherry or Banyuls vinegar

Sea salt and freshly ground pepper

20 small grape tomatoes

2 ounces Roquefort cheese, crumbled or finely diced

2 tablespoons sunflower seeds

1. Peel the carrots and beets and shred them separately with the shredding/grating disk of your food processor. Do the carrots first and there will be no need to rinse in between.
2. Rinse the spinach well and spin dry. Put the spinach in a large bowl and toss with the olive oil and sherry. Season with salt and pepper to taste.
3. Mound the spinach on 4 large plates. Top with a mound of shredded carrot and then a mound of shredded beet, arranging so that some of the carrot still shows through. Scatter 5 tomatoes around each plate.
4. Top with the Roquefort cheese and garnish with a sprinkling of sunflower seeds.

Main Dishes

Learning to plan a menu when you're new to eating mostly vegetarian can seem challenging at first, but it soon becomes second nature. You can always begin with a soup or salad. While pasta can be a first course or a main dish, we are counting it here as your primary dish. The same goes for the risottos. Pizza could be a lunch dish or light supper. And the polenta may count as a main dish but should be accompanied by steamed, roasted, or braised vegetables.

Many of the vegetable dishes in this chapter stand alone as a meal and need only some rice, quinoa, millet, or perhaps mashed or roasted potatoes to fill them out. When you're more comfortable with eating more vegetables and whole grains, you'll start composing your own menus, mixing and matching two or three dishes. An assortment of really tasty vegetarian burgers is included here, and just like the meaty kind, they are more fun when accompanied by a selection of "sides."

Keeping in mind that Dr. Rau's Maintenance Diet for Life allows you chicken or fish several times a week, we've included a selection of those to give you an idea of how to combine small amounts of chicken and fish with lots of vegetables for a nutritionally balanced meal that's not over-loaded with excess protein.

Look also to "The Salad Bar" section for an enticing variety of recipes that can serve as starter salads or main courses at lunch.

Pasta, Pizza, Risotto, and Polenta
Pasta with Broccoli Rabe and Feta Cheese
Pasta Primavera
    Creamy Tomato Sauce
Pasta with Tofu Pesto
Vegetable Lasagna
Cold Sesame Noodles
Instant Goat Cheese Pizzas with Arugula and Olives
Asparagus Risotto
Almost No-Stir Butternut Squash Risotto
Creamy Polenta with Manchego Cheese
    Baked Polenta

Vegetable and Grain Main Dishes and Some Sides
Asparagus Stir-Fry with Swiss Chard and Carrots
Quinoa-Stuffed Eggplant
Sesame Quinoa with Bok Choy and Shiitake Mushrooms
Eggplant Steaks with Sun-Dried Tomatoes and Olives
Fennel Gratin
Braised Kale with Carrots and Potatoes
Lentils with Goat Cheese and Sun-Dried Tomatoes
Roesti with Mixed Vegetables
    Steamed Mixed Vegetables
Potato Pie
    Flaky Pastry
    Olive Oil–Steamed Spinach
Twice-Baked Potatoes with Blue Cheese and Broccoli

Caramelized Sweet Potatoes and Beets with Green Beans and Toasted
  Pumpkin Seeds
Stuffed Sweet Dumpling Squash
Ginger-Lemon Tofu Steaks
Vegetarian Spring Rolls with Ginger-Sesame Dipping Sauce
Easy Vegetarian Chili with Bulgur and Pinto Beans
Moroccan Vegetable Stew
12-Minute Ratatouille
Succotash with Corn, Zucchini, and Green Beans
Zucchini Lasagna
Stuffed Giant Zucchini

Burgers and Patties
Amaranth Burgers
Barley and Black-Eyed Pea Cakes
Black Bean Burgers with Cashews and Carrots
Lentil and Quinoa Burgers
Curried Vegetable Patties

Chicken, Turkey, and Fish
Chicken and Vegetable Curry
Ginger Chicken Stir-Fry with Carrots, Snow Peas, and Red Pepper
Almost Meatless Shepherd's Pie
   Creamy Mashed Potatoes
Asian-Flavor Cod Baked with Napa Cabbage
Pecan-Crusted Catfish Fillets
   Pineapple Slaw

PASTA, PIZZA, RISOTTO, AND POLENTA

Pasta with Broccoli Rabe and Feta Cheese

Use spelt pasta or an imported semolina pasta from a good producer.

■ 4 SERVINGS

> 1 large bunch of broccoli rabe
>
> ½ pound gemelli (pasta twists), bow ties, or penne
>
> 4 tablespoons extra virgin olive oil
>
> 2 garlic cloves, thinly sliced
>
> 2 or 3 shakes of crushed hot red pepper
>
> ¼ cup finely diced or coarsely crumbled feta cheese
>
> Sea salt and freshly ground pepper
>
> Grated Pecorino Romano cheese

1. Wash the broccoli rabe well; drain briefly. Trim off and discard the bottom ½ inch of the thick stems. Cut the remaining stems into ½-inch pieces and the leaves and flowers into 1-inch pieces.

2. In a large saucepan of boiling salted water, cook the pasta until just tender, 10 to 12 minutes. Scoop out and reserve 1 cup of the pasta cooking water. Drain the pasta into a colander.

3. Add 3 tablespoons of the olive oil to the saucepan. Add the garlic and hot pepper and cook over medium-low heat until the garlic just begins to color, about 2 minutes. Pour in ½ cup of the pasta cooking water and let it bubble up.

4. Add the broccoli rabe and raise the heat to medium. Cook, stirring, until the broccoli leaves wilt, about 2 minutes. Pour in the remaining ½ cup cooking water and cook, stirring often, until the broccoli rabe is tender but still bright green, 5 to 6 minutes.

5. Dump the pasta into the pot. Add the feta cheese and remaining 1 tablespoon olive oil. Stir to mix well. Remove from the heat. Season lightly with sea salt and generously with black pepper. Serve in pasta bowls. Pass a bowl of Pecorino Romano cheese on the side.

Pasta Primavera with Creamy Tomato Sauce

Steaming makes preparing the vegetables for this classic pasta very easy. It's nice to have a lot of variety, but you can simplify as much as you like. Just make sure you have a total of 3 cups of vegetables.

■ 4 SERVINGS

⅔ cup cut-up asparagus

⅔ cup broccoli or cauliflower florets

⅔ cup sliced zucchini

12 ounces pasta bow ties or small twists

Creamy Tomato Sauce (recipe follows)

1 cup frozen baby peas, thawed

Grated Pecorino Romano or Manchego cheese or a mixture of the two

1. Steam the asparagus, broccoli, and zucchini over boiling water until just tender, 2 to 3 minutes. Reserve the steaming liquid for the tomato sauce.

2. In a large pot of boiling salted water, cook the pasta until almost tender, about 10 minutes. Drain into a colander.

3. Return the pasta to the pot and add the Creamy Tomato Sauce. Toss to coat. Simmer for 2 minutes over very low heat. Add the steamed vegetables and the peas and toss for a minute over heat to warm through. Pass the cheese on the side.

Creamy Tomato Sauce

Isn't it nice you can still enjoy many of the good things in life even though you are following my diet to improve your health. This comforting soup goes upscale with a splash of white wine and cream.

▓ MAKES ABOUT 3 CUPS

> 1 can (14 ounces) organic plum tomatoes
>
> 3 tablespoons extra virgin olive oil
>
> 1 garlic clove, minced
>
> Dash of crushed hot red pepper, or more to taste
>
> 1 tablespoon tomato paste
>
> ¼ cup dry white wine
>
> 1 cup vegetable steaming liquid (reserved from the Pasta Primavera) or
>   vegetable broth
>
> ⅓ cup heavy cream or soy creamer
>
> Salt and freshly ground black pepper

1. Puree the tomatoes with their juices in a blender or food processor.
2. In a large nonreactive saucepan or flameproof casserole, heat the olive oil over medium heat. Add the garlic and hot pepper and cook for 2 minutes. Add the tomato paste and cook, stirring, for 1 minute longer. Pour in the wine and boil until reduced by half. Add the vegetable liquid and pureed tomatoes and simmer for 15 minutes.
3. Stir in the cream. Season with salt and black pepper to taste.

Pasta with Tofu Pesto

Soft tofu makes a healthy substitute for the large amounts of oil and cheese found in many traditional pestos.

■ 4 SERVINGS

1½ cups (packed) fresh basil leaves

⅓ cup silken tofu

3 tablespoons freshly grated Pecorino Romano cheese

3 tablespoons extra virgin olive oil

1 tablespoon pine nuts (pignoli)

1½ teaspoons fresh lemon juice

1 garlic clove, chopped

Sea salt

½ pound whole wheat, spelt, or rice spaghetti or linguine

1 cup shelled fresh or frozen edamame or peas

1. To make the pesto: In a blender or food processor, combine the basil, tofu, cheese, olive oil, pine nuts, lemon juice, and garlic. Process, stopping once or twice to scrape down the sides of the bowl, until a coarse paste forms. Scrape the pesto into a large serving bowl.

2. In a large saucepan of boiling salted water, cook the pasta until just tender, about 10 minutes or as the package directs. If using thawed frozen edamame or peas, add them directly to the bowl of pesto. If using fresh edamame or peas, add them to the pasta during the last 1 minute of cooking time.

3. Scoop out ½ cup of the pasta cooking water and add to the pesto. Drain the pasta (and fresh edamame) in a colander and turn into the bowl. Toss gently to coat with the pesto. Serve at once.

Vegetable Lasagna

No-cook noodles take much of the effort out of making lasagna, as do other convenience foods like frozen spinach and prepared sauces.

■ 6 SERVINGS

    1 medium head of cauliflower, separated into florets

    2 medium fennel bulbs, trimmed and halved

    3 cups of your favorite organic tomato or marinara sauce

    1 box (16 ounces) imported no-boil lasagna noodles, such as Barilla

    1 bag (12 ounces) frozen organic whole leaf spinach, thawed and
       squeezed to remove excess water

    1 cup grated Pecorino Romano cheese (about 3 ounces)

    3 tablespoons extra virgin olive oil

    Sea salt and freshly ground pepper

    3 ounces goat cheese or feta, crumbled (about 1 cup)

1. Preheat the oven to 325°F. Lightly oil an 8 × 11-inch baking dish.

2. Slice both the cauliflower florets and the fennel pieces into ¼-inch thick slices. Steam them over boiling water until just softened, 4 to 5 minutes.

3. To assemble the lasagna, ladle about ⅔ cup of the tomato sauce over the bottom of the baking dish. Arrange 3 sheets of the pasta, side by side, over the sauce to cover the dish completely. Spread half of the spinach evenly over the pasta. Sprinkle ⅓ cup of the Romano cheese evenly over the spinach. Then add a layer of half the cauliflower and half the fennel, alternating the vegetables. Drizzle 1½ tablespoons of the olive oil over the vegetables. Season with a sprinkling of sea salt and plenty of freshly ground pepper. Scatter half the goat cheese over the vegetables and top with ⅔ cup tomato sauce, spooning it to cover as much area as possible.

4. Make a second layer in similar fashion: Add another 3 sheets pasta over the sauce, pressing them down gently to fill up any spaces. Layer the remaining spinach, another ⅓ cup of the cheese, and the remaining veg-

etables. Drizzle with the remaining oil and a sprinkling of salt and pepper. Top with the remaining goat cheese and another ⅔ cup sauce. Finally, cover with the last 3 sheets of pasta, pressing lightly to help compact the lasagna. Spread the last of the sauce over them and sprinkle with the remaining Pecorino Romano cheese. Cover the dish with aluminum foil, tenting it so the foil does not come in contact with the tomato sauce. Either bake at once or cover and refrigerate for several hours.

5. When you're ready to cook the lasagna, preheat the oven to 350°F. Bake the lasagna, covered, for 25 to 30 minutes, until just heated through. Uncover and bake 10 minutes longer. Remove from the oven and let stand for about 10 minutes before cutting.

Cold Sesame Noodles

Spicy noodles are the perfect backdrop for an endless array of flavors, so feel free to toss in any leftover vegetables you may have on hand, such as lightly steamed asparagus, green beans, or broccoli.

▨ 4 SERVINGS

⅓ cup natural cashew butter

2 tablespoons organic wheat-free soy tamari

2 tablespoons toasted sesame oil

1 tablespoon minced fresh ginger

2 teaspoons unseasoned rice vinegar or fresh lime juice

1 garlic clove, crushed through a press

2 or 3 shakes of crushed hot red pepper, or to taste

1 cucumber

½ pound whole wheat spaghetti or linguine

Sea salt (optional)

1 medium-large carrot, peeled and shredded

1 tablespoon minced fresh chives

1 tablespoon toasted sesame seeds

1. In a large bowl, mix together the cashew butter, tamari, sesame oil, ginger, rice vinegar, garlic, and crushed hot pepper. Set the sesame sauce aside.

2. Peel the cucumber and cut in half lengthwise. Scrape out the seeds with a small spoon. Cut cucumber crosswise into diagonal slices about ¼-inch thick.

3. In a large saucepan of boiling salted water, cook the pasta until just tender, about 10 minutes or as the package directs. Scoop out ⅓ cup of the pasta cooking water and add to the sesame sauce, stirring until well blended. Taste, adding a dash of salt if needed. Drain the pasta in a colander and rinse under cold running water until cool; drain again. Add the pasta, cucumber, carrot, and chives to the sauce. Toss gently to coat. Serve with the sesame seeds sprinkled on top.

Instant Goat Cheese Pizzas with Arugula and Olives

You can enjoy healthful pizza anytime you want, using tortillas as the base. Vary toppings as you like. Fresh tomatoes, basil, and shaved Manchego cheese are other nice options.

■ SERVES 4 TO 6

> 2 large (11- to 12-inch) sprouted wheat or whole wheat flour tortillas
>
> ⅓ cup extra virgin olive oil
>
> 4 ounces fresh white goat cheese
>
> 1 cup chopped pitted Kalamata olives, or any pitted olives
>
> 2 cups lightly packed baby arugula or spinach leaves

1. Preheat the oven to 475°F. Lightly brush the tortillas with 1½ tablespoons of the olive oil, place on baking sheets, and bake until the tortillas just begin to crisp, about 2 minutes. Turn the tortillas over and

brush the tortillas with another 1½ tablespoons olive oil and sprinkle half the goat cheese and half the olives over each. Bake for 3 to 5 minutes.

2. Scatter the arugula or spinach on top and drizzle with the remaining olive oil. Return to the oven and bake the pizzas for 1 to 2 minutes, until heated through.

Asparagus Risotto

While vegetables are lovely cooked until just tender, when they are blended into a risotto they are usually cooked fully soft so that they blend with the sauce. Here the asparagus stalks are cooked the entire time with the rice, but the tips are added near the end to retain their texture.

4 TO 6 SERVINGS

1 large bunch of asparagus, 1 to 1¼ pounds
2 tablespoons extra virgin olive oil
¼ cup thinly sliced leek (white and pale green)
1 cup Arborio rice
1 teaspoon chopped fresh tarragon leaves or crumbled dried
¼ cup dry white wine
4 to 5 cups hot vegetable or chicken broth
2 tablespoons unsalted butter
⅓ cup grated Manchego cheese
Sea salt and freshly ground pepper

1. Cut off the whitish bottom parts of the asparagus stalks. Cut the remaining green stalks into thin rounds, stopping about 1 inch from the tips. Cut the tips lengthwise in half and set aside.
2. In a large heavy saucepan, heat the olive oil over medium heat. Add the leek and cook, stirring once or twice, for 2 minutes. Add the rice and tarragon and cook, stirring often, for 2 minutes longer.
3. Pour in the wine and cook, stirring, until most of it evaporates. Add

the sliced asparagus stalks and ⅔ cup of the warm broth and continue to cook, stirring occasionally, until most of the liquid is absorbed. Add ½ cup broth and cook, stirring often, until most of the liquid is absorbed. Continue to cook, gradually adding more broth about ½ cup at a time, for 10 minutes.

4. Add the asparagus tips and continue to cook in the same manner, adding more broth as needed, until the rice is al dente and the sauce around it is thicky and creamy, 8 to 10 minutes longer.

5. Stir in the butter and cheese. Season lightly with salt and generously with pepper. Serve at once.

Almost No-Stir Butternut Squash Risotto

■ 4 TO 6 SERVINGS

2 tablespoons extra virgin olive oil

¼ cup thinly sliced leek (white and pale green)

1 cup Arborio rice

2½ cups diced (½-inch) organic butternut squash

½ teaspoon freshly grated nutmeg

4½ cups heated vegetable broth

2 tablespoons unsalted butter

Sea salt and freshly ground pepper

1. Heat the olive oil in a large heavy saucepan over medium heat. Add the leek and cook until softened, about 2 minutes. Add the rice and cook for 2 minutes, stirring frequently.

2. Add the squash, nutmeg, and broth. Stir to mix. Bring to a boil, reduce the heat to low, cover, and cook until the squash is tender, most of the liquid has been absorbed, and the risotto has the consistency of a thick soup, 18 to 20 minutes.

3. Stir in the butter and season with salt and pepper.

Creamy Polenta with Manchego Cheese

Polenta *is simply the Italian word for cornmeal or grits. Like any whole grain, it is best fresh and ideally should be stored in the refrigerator or freezer. Whether you serve this as a main course with fresh tomato sauce or as a side with an assortment of steamed vegetables, it offers a delightful alternative to pasta or rice.*

■ 6 SERVINGS

1 cup polenta stone-ground yellow cornmeal

1 teaspoon sea salt

Dash of cayenne

½ cup heavy cream

2 tablespoons unsalted butter

⅓ cup shredded Manchego cheese

1. In a medium bowl, stir together the cornmeal with 2 cups of water. Bring another 2 cups of water with the salt and cayenne to a boil in a heavy saucepan over medium heat.

2. Gradually stir the cornmeal slurry into the boiling water. Reduce the heat to medium–low and continue to cook, stirring often, for 20 minutes. Stir in ¼ cup of the cream and continue to cook, stirring, until the polenta thickens and begins to pull away from the sides of the pan. If the liquid evaporates too quickly, add more water.

3. When the polenta is thick and the cornmeal is tender, remove from the heat. Stir in the rest of the cream, the butter, and the cheese. Serve at once.

VARIATION BAKED POLENTA: Prepare the polenta as directed above. Turn out into a buttered baking dish, spread out into a ½-inch layer, and let cool until set. (The firm polenta can be refrigerated overnight.) Then cut into rounds or squares and bake in a 425°F oven until lightly browned on top and heated through, 10 to 15 minutes.

VEGETABLE AND GRAIN MAIN DISHES AND SOME SIDES

Asparagus Stir-Fry
with Swiss Chard and Carrots

Here's a satisfying colorful stir-fry you can throw together in 15 minutes or less. Serve with steamed basmati rice.

■ 3 TO 4 SERVINGS

1 small bunch of Swiss chard

2 tablespoons extra virgin olive oil

¾ pound asparagus, cut into 1-inch lengths

2 medium carrots, peeled and sliced on the diagonal

2 teaspoons minced fresh ginger

⅔ cup vegetable or chicken broth

1 tablespoon organic wheat-free tamari

2 teaspoons cornstarch

1 tablespoon Asian sesame oil

¼ cup roasted cashews

1. Rinse the chard well. Cut the green leaves off the white stems. Shred the leaves and set aside. Cut the stems in half lengthwise if they are thick, then cut crosswise into ¾-inch slices.
2. Heat the olive oil in a wok or large skillet. Add the asparagus, carrots, and ginger and sauté for 1 to 2 minutes. Add the chard stems and ⅓ cup of the broth. Cover, reduce the heat to medium, and cook for 3 minutes.
3. Meanwhile, combine the remaining broth with the tamari. Stir in the cornstarch. Add to the wok and bring to a boil, tossing until the vegetables are evenly coated and the sauce is thickened, about 1 minute.
4. Transfer to a platter. Drizzle the sesame oil over the stir-fry and sprinkle the cashews on top.

Quinoa-Stuffed Eggplant

Quinoa is a great grain, rich in essential amino acids. It has a fine, nutty taste, but must be rinsed before using to wash off its slightly bitter coating. To do so, rinse in a bowl of warm water and drain in a sieve two or three times before using.

■ 4 SERVINGS

4 Japanese eggplants (long skinny, light purple ones)

2½ tablespoons extra virgin olive oil

½ cup quinoa

2 large ripe plum tomatoes, peeled, seeded, and finely diced

2 tablespoons fresh lemon juice

2 tablespoons pine nuts (pignoli)

1 garlic clove, minced

1 small fennel bulb, finely diced

1 tablespoon chopped fresh basil or 1 teaspoon dried oregano

Sea salt and freshly ground pepper

½ cup shredded Pecorino Romano cheese

1. Preheat the oven to 375°F. Trim off the eggplant stems and slice the eggplants in half lengthwise; brush lightly with ½ tablespoon olive oil and place face down on a baking sheet. Bake for 20 minutes, or until just tender.

2. Meanwhile, rinse the quinoa several times. Place in a small saucepan with 1 cup lightly salted water, cover, and cook for 12 to 15 minutes, until the liquid is absorbed and the quinoa is tender.

3. As soon as the eggplants are cool enough to handle, use a large spoon to gently scoop out the centers, leaving a ¼-inch shell. Be careful not to tear the skin. Coarsely chop the eggplant and put it in a mixing bowl. Add the tomatoes and lemon juice and mix well.

4. In a medium skillet, combine 2 tablespoons of the olive oil with the pine nuts and garlic. Set over medium heat and cook, stirring, for

2 minutes. Add the fennel and continue to cook, stirring often, until it softens, about 3 minutes longer. Add the fennel mixture to the eggplant along with the quinoa and basil; stir to blend. Season with salt and pepper to taste.

5. Fill the eggplant shells with the vegetable mixture. Top with the shredded cheese and place in a baking dish. The recipe can be prepared ahead to this point. Set aside at room temperature for up to 2 hours or refrigerate for up to 6 hours. (If refrigerated, return to room temperature before baking.)

6. When ready to serve, place the stuffed eggplants in a 375°F oven and bake for 7 to 10 minutes, until the vegetables are heated through and the cheese is melted.

Sesame Quinoa with Bok Choy and Shiitake Mushrooms

Quinoa is an excellent grain, both nutritious and delicious. Here it is combined with Asian flavors for a main course that is pleasing in both taste and texture. Serve with steamed carrots.

■ 4 SERVINGS

1 cup quinoa

2 tablespoons extra virgin olive oil

1 teaspoon minced fresh ginger

6 ounces fresh shiitake mushrooms, stems removed, caps thinly sliced

1 pound bok choy, trimmed and sliced ½ inch thick (white stems and
    green leaves)

1 tablespoon Asian sesame oil

Pinch of sea salt

1 tablespoon toasted sesame seeds

1. Put the quinoa in a medium bowl and fill with warm water. Swish the quinoa around with your fingers, then drain into a sieve. Repeat the rinsing and draining 2 more times.

2. In a medium saucepan, bring 2 cups lightly salted water to a boil. Add the quinoa, give it a stir, reduce the heat to low, cover, and cook for 12 to 15 minutes, until the quinoa is tender and has opened up so you can see its little "halos."

3. Heat the olive oil in a large skillet over medium-high heat. Add the ginger, mushrooms, and bok choy. Sauté, stirring often, for about 3 minutes, until the bok choy is just tender.

4. Remove from the heat, add the quinoa, and toss to combine the grain with the vegetables. Drizzle on the sesame oil and mix well. Season with salt to taste. Sprinkle the sesame seeds on top.

Eggplant Steaks with Sun-Dried Tomatoes and Olives

Serve with pasta, polenta, or rice. Accompany with steamed broccoli or braised escarole or kale.

▨ 4 SERVINGS

2 medium-large eggplants (about 1 pound each)

Coarse sea salt

6 tablespoons extra virgin olive oil

⅓ cup crumbled goat cheese or sheep's milk feta

8 sun-dried tomato halves packed in olive oil, drained and coarsely chopped

12 pitted Kalamata olives, coarsely chopped

¼ cup grated Pecorino Romano cheese

2 to 3 tablespoons slivered fresh basil leaves, for garnish

1. Trim the ends from the eggplants and peel off the skin. Cut each eggplant lengthwise into four or more ½-inch-thick slices. (Some of the slices will be smaller than others, but all should be of equal thickness.) If needed, trim a thin slice from each of the rounded sides so the pieces will lie flat on the baking sheet. Sprinkle the slices with coarse salt and layer in a colander to drain for at least 30 minutes or for up to 2 hours. Rinse the eggplant slices under cold running water and dry well with paper towels, pressing to remove as much moisture as possible.

2. Preheat the broiler and position the oven rack about 4 inches from the heat. Line a large heavy baking sheet with aluminum foil. Arrange the eggplant slices on the sheet in a single layer and brush both sides with oil. Broil for 7 to 9 minutes, turning once, until the eggplant is tender and lightly browned on both sides. Leave the broiler on.

3. Meanwhile, combine the goat cheese, sun-dried tomatoes, and olives in a small bowl. Toss gently to mix. Divide the mixture evenly over the broiled eggplant slices. Sprinkle the Pecorino Romano cheese evenly over each slice and return to the oven. Broil for 1 minute, or until the goat cheese has softened and the grated cheese is just beginning to brown at the edges. Watch carefully to avoid burning. Scatter basil over the top of each slice and serve at once.

Fennel Gratin

Broiling the fennel first brings out its lovely nutty flavor. This can easily serve as the centerpiece of a vegetarian plate or as a side dish to offer with chicken or fish.

■ 4 SERVINGS

2 bulbs of fennel, trimmed and cut lengthwise into ⅜-inch slices

3 tablespoons extra virgin olive oil

Sea salt and freshly ground pepper

1 cup vegetable or chicken broth

1 cup fresh spelt, whole-grain, or whole wheat bread crumbs

¼ cup freshly grated Pecorino Romano cheese

1 teaspoon fennel seeds, crushed

1. Preheat the broiler. Using 2 tablespoons of the olive oil, brush both sides of the fennel slices. Arrange in a single layer on a baking sheet and season lightly with salt and pepper.

2. Broil the fennel slices about 4 inches from the heat, turning once, until they are lightly colored, about 3 minutes per side. Transfer the fennel to a gratin or flameproof baking dish, overlapping the slices as necessary to fit. Reduce the oven temperature to 400°F.

3. Pour the broth over the fennel, cover with foil, and bake for 10 to 15 minutes, until the fennel is tender but still firm and most of the liquid is absorbed.

4. Combine the bread crumbs, cheese, and fennel seeds. Turn the fennel slices over and sprinkle the seasoned bread crumbs on top. Drizzle with the remaining 1 tablespoon olive oil. Return to the oven and bake uncovered for 5 to 7 minutes longer, or until the fennel is tender and the crumb topping is lightly browned.

Braised Kale with Carrots and Potatoes

You'll be surprised how savory and satisfying this simple vegetable stew is. Serve with quinoa, millet, or steamed rice.

■ 3 TO 4 SERVINGS

1 large bunch of kale, preferably lacinato kale

3 tablespoons extra virgin olive oil

1 small leek (white and pale green), thinly sliced

¾ to 1 cup vegetable or chicken broth

2 medium carrots, peeled and roll-cut into ½-inch triangles or thickly sliced

2 medium Yukon gold potatoes, peeled and cut into ½- to ¾-inch cubes

Sea salt and freshly ground pepper

1. Strip the thick stems off the kale leaves. Cut the leaves crosswise into ¼-inch strips.

2. In a large saucepan or flameproof casserole, heat the olive oil over medium heat. Add the leek, and cook until softened, about 3 minutes.

3. Add the kale in 2 or 3 handfuls, stirring to wilt. Add the broth and bring to a boil. Reduce the heat to low, cover, and simmer for 10 minutes.

4. Add the carrots and potatoes, cover, and simmer until the potatoes are tender, about 10 minutes. Season with salt and pepper before serving.

Lentils with Goat Cheese and Sun-Dried Tomatoes

You can make this recipe with regular greenish brown lentils or with the tiny dark lentils de Puy, which hold their shape very nicely and cook a little quicker. Either way, offer the dish warm as a vegetable main course or at room temperature as a salad.

■ 4 TO 6 SERVINGS

2 medium carrots, peeled and chopped

2 celery ribs, chopped

2 garlic cloves, chopped

3 tablespoons extra virgin olive oil

1 cup lentils

1 bay leaf

1 whole clove

¼ cup chopped fresh parsley

¼ cup diced oil-packed sun-dried tomatoes

1 tablespoon wine vinegar

Sea salt and freshly ground pepper

2 ounces fresh white goat cheese

1. In a large saucepan or flameproof casserole, cook the carrots, celery, and garlic in 2 tablespoons of the olive oil over medium heat, stirring occasionally, until the vegetables soften slightly, 2 to 3 minutes.
2. Add the lentils, bay leaf, clove, and 2 tablespoons of the parsley. Pour in enough water to just cover. Bring to a boil, reduce the heat, and simmer partially covered, until the liquid is almost all evaporated and the lentils are tender but still hold their shape, 25 to 35 minutes. If the pan becomes dry, add a little water ⅓ cup at a time.
3. Stir in the sun-dried tomatoes and vinegar. Season with sea salt and pepper to taste.
4. Fish out and discard the bay leaf and clove. Transfer the lentils to a serving bowl and stir in the goat cheese, cut into bits, along with the remaining 1 tablespoon olive oil. Serve warm or at room temperature.

Roesti with Mixed Vegetables

Roesti is one of the great Swiss dishes. Russet, or baking potatoes, are boiled in their skins, chilled to set the starch, and then grated the next day. The shredded potato is fried in a large flat cake until golden brown. Served by itself, with vegetables, or with anything you like, it makes a marvelous lunch or supper. Try it with a nice green salad.

■ 4 SERVINGS

4 large baking potatoes, about 10 ounces each
1 teaspoon coarse sea salt
¼ teaspoon freshly ground pepper
½ cup plus 2 tablespoons extra virgin olive oil
4 teaspoons unsalted butter
Steamed Mixed Vegetables (recipe follows)

1. Steam the whole potatoes in their skins until they are tender all the way through when pierced with the tip of a small knife, 30 to 40

minutes. Check the water in your steamer about halfway through to see if it needs replenishing. Let the potatoes cool, then refrigerate overnight.

2.   The next day, peel the potatoes. The skins should slip right off. Finely shred the potatoes on the coarse grating disk of your food processor or on the large holes of a box or flat grater. Toss the shredded potato with the salt and pepper.

3.   Heat 1½ tablespoons of the olive oil in a heavy 6½- to 7-inch skillet over medium-high heat. Pick up ¼ of the potatoes with your hand and drop in the center of the skillet in a mound. Flatten evenly with a wide spatula to make a cake about ⅜ inch thick. Reduce the heat slightly and fry the roesti until golden brown on the bottom, 5 to 7 minutes. Carefully set a plate over the skillet and invert the roesti onto the plate. Heat another 1 tablespoon olive oil in the skillet and slide the roesti back into the pan to brown the second side. When it is just about done, dot the sides of the pan with 1 teaspoon of the butter and tilt to distribute the melted butter. Slide the roesti onto a platter and keep hot in a low oven while you repeat three more times with the remaining ingredients.

4.   Place a hot roesti on each of 4 warmed dinner plates. Spoon the vegetables around the potato cakes.

Steamed Mixed Vegetables

You can use any assortment of vegetables you like here, depending on what is fresh and in the market. You want to end up with about 4 cups.

■ 4 SERVINGS

4 ounces thin green beans, trimmed

2 medium carrots, peeled and thickly sliced on an angle

8 asparagus spears, cut into 1-inch lengths

1 medium zucchini, trimmed and sliced on an angle

1½ tablespoons fresh lemon juice

1½ tablespoons extra virgin olive oil

Coarse sea salt and freshly ground pepper

1. Arrange the green beans and carrots on the rack of a steamer in separate piles over plenty of boiling salted water. Cover and steam until tender, 4 to 5 minutes. Remove to a platter.

2. Add the asparagus and zucchini to the steamer and cook until just tender, 2 to 3 minutes. Add to the platter.

3. Sprinkle the lemon juice and olive oil over the vegetables and toss lightly. Season with salt and pepper to taste.

Potato Pie

Forget everything you ever thought about carbohydrates. Many of them are good for you, especially potatoes. This irresistible pie, actually a lovely double-crust tart, is beautiful and makes a fabulous star attraction for luncheon or dinner. Begin with a nice Dr. Rau salad and serve Olive Oil–Steamed Spinach (page 252) or a colorful assortment of steamed or roasted vegetables on the side.

■ 8 SERVINGS

Flaky Pastry (recipe follows)

1 teaspoon Dijon mustard

2 pounds Yukon gold or waxy heirloom potatoes

¼ cup thinly sliced leek (white and pale green)

2 tablespoons chopped fresh parsley

4 tablespoons unsalted butter, melted

½ cup shredded Manchego cheese

Coarse sea salt and freshly ground pepper

¼ teaspoon freshly grated nutmeg

1 tablespoon egg wash (reserved from Flaky Pastry)

6 tablespoons heavy cream

1. Prepare and chill the Flaky Pastry as directed on page 251. Roll out the larger pastry disk to a round about ⅛ inch thick. Fit without stretching into a 9-inch tart pan with a removable bottom. Prick the pastry all over with a fork and paint lightly with the mustard. Chill while you prepare the filling.

2. Preheat the oven to 400°F. Peel the potatoes, and with a large sharp knife or a mandolin, slice them very thinly. Put the potato slices in a bowl and toss with the leek, parsley, and 2 tablespoons of the melted butter.

3. Sprinkle about 2 tablespoons of the cheese over the bottom of the pastry shell. Arrange half the potato slices in the pastry shell, beginning at the outer edge and overlapping the slices in concentric circles. Season with half the nutmeg and salt and pepper to taste. Sprinkle 3 tablespoons of the cheese over the potatoes. Repeat with a second layer, using the rest of the potatoes, cheese, and nutmeg. Season again with salt and pepper. Drizzle the remaining melted butter over the top.

4. Roll out the smaller pastry disk and set it on top of the pie. Trim the edges of both sheets of pastry to ½ inch. Fold over and crimp. Press a rolling pin over the edges of the pan to trim evenly. With the tip of a small knife or a ½-inch plain pastry tip, cut out a small circle in the center of the pie to act as a steam vent. Brush the top of the pie with the reserved egg wash.

5. Bake for 50 minutes, or until the pie is golden brown and the potatoes are tender. Remove from the oven and let stand for 10 minutes. Then, using a funnel, pour half the cream into the hole in the center of the pie. Using mitts to protect your hands, lift the hot pan and slowly tilt it around slightly in all directions to distribute the cream. Repeat with the remaining cream. Let the pie stand for 10 to 15 minutes before serving.

Flaky Pastry

■ MAKES A 9-INCH DOUBLE CRUST

1¾ cups spelt pastry flour

¼ teaspoon baking powder

⅛ teaspoon fine sea salt

1 small egg, beaten with 2 teaspoons water

¼ cup sunflower oil

1. In a large bowl, combine the flour, baking powder, and salt. Whisk gently to blend.
2. Spoon out 1 tablespoon of the beaten egg and water to use as glaze in step 4 of the Potato Pie recipe (page 250).
3. In a small bowl, whisk together the remaining beaten egg, the oil, and ⅓ cup ice cold water. With a large fork, toss the flour mixture while you sprinkle the liquid over the dough. Continue to mix with the fork until the dough just comes together. If necessary, sprinkle on a little extra water, 1 tablespoon at a time, to make a cohesive but not sticky dough.
4. Press the dough together into a ball with your hands. Divide into 2 portions, one a bit larger than the other. Roll these lightly into balls and flatten into 2 disks. Dust with a little more flour to prevent sticking and wrap in plastic or waxed paper. Refrigerate the dough for 30 to 60 minutes before rolling out.

Olive Oil–Steamed Spinach

After cooking, spinach is hard to season evenly. By tossing with the oil, salt, and pepper before steaming, the leaves both taste better and maintain their integrity. Do not overcook.

■ 2 TO 3 SERVINGS

> 1 pound washed baby spinach
>
> 2 tablespoons extra virgin olive oil
>
> Sea salt and freshly ground pepper

1. Set up a large pot of boiling water with a steamer insert. Place the spinach in a large bowl. Toss with the olive oil and salt and pepper to taste.
2. Transfer the seasoned spinach to the steamer and cook the spinach for about 3 minutes, until just wilted. Serve at once.

Twice-Baked Potatoes with Blue Cheese and Broccoli

The organisms that give Roquefort and other similar cheeses their distinctive blue veins are good for your digestive tract. And even a small amount adds wonderful flavor to many foods. Half of one of these overstuffed potatoes makes a satisfying main dinner, especially when paired with an assortment of other vegetables, such as steamed carrots and Marinated Roasted Beets (page 219).

■ 2 SERVINGS

> 1 large baking potato (10 to 12 ounces), scrubbed
>
> 1 cup broccoli florets
>
> 1½ tablespoons unsalted butter

¾ ounce Roquefort cheese, crumbled (about 2 tablespoons)

2 to 3 tablespoons soy, rice, or goat milk

Sea salt and freshly ground black pepper to taste

½ ounce Manchego cheese, in one piece

1. Preheat the oven to 400°F. Prick the potato in 2 places with the tip of a small knife. Put the potato right on the rack and bake for 1 hour, or until the skin is crisp and the potato is very tender. Leave the oven on.

2. While the potato is baking, steam the broccoli for 1½ to 2 minutes, until it is just tender but still bright green. Coarsely chop half of the largest florets.

3. Cut the hot baked potato in half lengthwise, using a mitt if necessary to protect your hands. Scoop the potato into a bowl; set the skins aside. Mash the hot baked potato with the butter and Roquefort cheese. Mix in enough of the milk to make the potato creamy. Fold in the chopped broccoli. Season with salt and pepper to taste.

4. Mound the potato-broccoli mixture in the potato skins. Press the remaining broccoli into the top. Shave the Manchego cheese over the broccoli to cover it with a very thin layer. Return to the oven for 5 to 10 minutes, until the filling is hot and the cheese on top is melted.

Caramelized Sweet Potatoes and Beets with Green Beans and Toasted Pumpkin Seeds

This colorful dish makes a beautiful presentation, especially in the fall and winter months. A cast-iron skillet works best but a stainless steel frying pan will do.

■ 4 SERVINGS

3 tablespoons pumpkin seeds

2 medium beets, peeled and cut into ⅜- to ½-inch dice

½ pound thin green beans, trimmed

4 tablespoons extra virgin olive oil

2 small sweet potatoes, peeled and cut into ⅜- to ½-inch dice

Juice of ½ lemon

Salt and freshly ground pepper

2 tablespoons balsamic vinegar

1. In a dry medium skillet, toast the pumpkin seeds over medium heat until fragrant and lightly browned, about 3 minutes. Set aside.

2. Steam the beets until tender, 10 to 15 minutes. Steam the green beans until tender, 4 to 5 minutes.

3. Meanwhile, in a large heavy skillet, heat 2 tablespoons of the olive oil over medium-high heat. Add the sweet potatoes and sauté, tossing, until lightly browned, about 5 minutes. Pour ⅓ cup water into the skillet, cover, reduce the heat to low, and cook until the sweet potatoes are just tender, 5 to 7 minutes longer. Mound in the center of a platter.

4. Heat 1 tablespoon of the oil in the skillet and add the green beans. Toss over medium-high heat for 1 to 2 minutes to reheat. Drizzle with the lemon juice. Season with salt and pepper to taste. Arrange the beans around the sweet potatoes.

5. Heat the remaining 1 tablespoon of oil in the same skillet. Add the balsamic vinegar and cook until reduced by half, 30 to 60 seconds. Add the beets and toss to coat with the dressing. Spoon the dressed beets over the sweet potatoes. Sprinkle the toasted pumpkin seeds on top.

Stuffed Sweet Dumpling Squash

In summer and early fall, when farmers' markets are filled with produce and even the supermarkets stock locally grown vegetables, you'll be sure to see these sweet, small squash. Partially baked until soft enough to carve, the little squashes are filled with cracked wheat, vegetables, and dried currants all bound in a sweetly spiced tomato sauce. They make a charming presentation.

NOTE: If you are intolerant of wheat, substitute cooked quinoa for the bulgur and skip step 2.

■ 4 SERVINGS

> 4 small squash, such as Sweet Dumpling (about 6 ounces each)
> 1 cup bulgur
> 1 large Yukon gold potato, peeled and halved
> 1 large parsnip, peeled and halved
> 2 medium carrots, peeled and halved
> 3 tablespoons extra virgin olive oil
> ⅓ cup chopped leek (white and pale green)
> 1 cup shredded kale
> ¼ cup currants or coarsely chopped raisins
> ½ cup tomato sauce
> ½ teaspoon ground cinnamon
> Sea salt and cayenne

1. Preheat the oven to 375°F. Wash the squash well, dry, and arrange in a lightly oiled baking dish. Bake for 25 to 30 minutes, or until the squash are tender but still firm.
2. Meanwhile, soak the bulgur in warm water to cover until softened, 20 to 30 minutes. Drain well.
3. Steam the potato, parsnip, and carrots until just tender; reserve the steaming liquid. Let the vegetables cool; then cut into fine dice.

4. In a large skillet, heat the olive oil over medium heat. Add the leek and cook until softened, about 3 minutes. Add the kale and cook, stirring, until wilted. Add ¾ cup of the steaming liquid. Bring to a boil, reduce the heat, cover, and cook until the kale is almost tender, 10 to 15 minutes.

5. Add the diced potato, parsnip, and carrots, the currants, tomato sauce, and cinnamon. Season lightly with salt and cayenne. Simmer uncovered, stirring often, for 10 minutes, or until the kale is tender. Stir in the bulgur and season with more salt and cayenne to taste. If the mixture is dry, add a little more steaming liquid.

6. Cut the tops off the squash as you would a jack-o'-lantern. Scoop out the seeds and membranes. Fill the squash with the vegetable and bulgur mixture and set the tops back in place. (The recipe can be prepared ahead to this point.) When ready to serve, return to a 375°F oven for 10 to 15 minutes to reheat.

Ginger-Lemon Tofu Steaks

Here the bland flavor of tofu is enlivened with a marinade of fresh ginger, lemon, and balsamic vinegar. Serve with rice and steamed broccoli florets.

■ 2 SERVINGS

½ pound extra-firm tofu

4 tablespoons extra virgin olive oil

2 teaspoons minced fresh ginger

1 garlic clove, minced

Dash of crushed hot red pepper

1 tablespoon balsamic vinegar

1 tablespoon organic wheat-free tamari

Grated zest and juice from ½ large lemon

Sea salt and freshly ground black pepper

1. Cut the tofu into ½-inch-thick slabs. Drain between several thicknesses of paper towels with a heavy tray on top to press out as much water as possible.

2. In a heavy skillet, heat half the olive oil over medium heat until very hot. Add the tofu steaks and fry, turning once with a wide spatula, until lightly browned and crispy on both sides, about 5 minutes. Drain on paper towels. Pour off any excess oil and carefully wipe out the pan with paper towels.

3. Heat the remaining oil in the skillet over medium-low heat. Add the ginger, garlic, and hot pepper and cook until fragrant but not browned, 2 to 3 minutes. Pour in the vinegar, tamari, and ¼ cup water. Boil until reduced by half. Stir in the lemon zest and lemon juice. Season lightly with salt and generously with black pepper.

4. Add the tofu steaks to the skillet, reduce the heat to low, and simmer, turning once, until the steaks are hot and almost all the marinade has been absorbed, 3 to 5 minutes.

Vegetarian Spring Rolls with Ginger-Sesame Dipping Sauce
■ 4 SERVINGS

    1 cup shredded spinach, well rinsed

    1 cup finely shredded cabbage

    1 cup shredded carrot

    ½ cup shredded daikon

    1 tablespoon fresh lime juice or rice vinegar

    1 tablespoon sunflower oil

    4 round sheets of rice paper

    Ginger-Sesame Dipping Sauce (recipe follows)

1. In a large bowl, toss the spinach, cabbage, carrot, and daikon with the lime juice and oil, trying to keep the shreds going in the same direction as much as possible.

2. One at a time, dip a rice paper wrapper in a bowl of warm water until it is soft, 20 to 30 seconds, or slightly longer if the wrappers have been on the shelf for a while. Remove, letting the extra water run back into the bowl and set flat on a sheet of waxed paper.

3. Place about one-fourth of the vegetables in the center of the wrapper. Fold up the bottom and sides and roll up as you would an egg roll. (The spring rolls can be assembled up to 3 hours in advance, covered, and refrigerated.)

4. To serve, cut the rolls in half and serve with small bowls of Ginger-Sesame Dipping Sauce.

Ginger-Sesame Dipping Sauce

3 tablespoons organic wheat-free tamari

2 tablespoons Asian sesame oil

2 tablespoons rice vinegar

1 garlic clove, finely minced

1 teaspoon grated fresh ginger

½ teaspoon raw brown sugar

Combine all the ingredients. Stir to dissolve the brown sugar.

Easy Vegetarian Chili
with Bulgur and Pinto Beans

There are a lot of ingredients here, but really not much work. Texture is an important part of vegetarian cooking and the bulgur, which retains some bite, offers a pleasing contrast to the soft vegetables. Serve, if you like, with plain goat yogurt, baked tortilla chips, shredded Manchego cheese, and pickled jalapeño peppers on the side.

■ 6 TO 8 SERVINGS

    2 celery ribs, chopped

    ¼ cup extra virgin olive oil

    2 garlic cloves, finely chopped

    1½ tablespoons ancho chile powder

    2 teaspoons ground cumin

    ½ teaspoon ground cinnamon

    2 carrots, peeled and coarsely chopped

    ½ head of cabbage, coarsely chopped

    ½ head of cauliflower, coarsely chopped

    1 teaspoon coarse sea salt

    1 can (14½ ounces) diced tomatoes, with their juices

    2 cups vegetable or chicken broth

    1 medium zucchini, coarsely chopped

    ¾ cup bulgur

    1 can (15 ounces) pinto beans, rinsed and drained

1. In a large flameproof casserole, cook the celery in the olive oil over medium heat for 5 minutes. Add the garlic and cook, stirring, for 2 minutes. Add the chile powder, cumin, and cinnamon and cook, stirring, for 1 minute longer to toast the spices.

2. Add the carrots, cabbage, cauliflower, and salt. Stir to coat the vegetables with the spiced oil. Add the tomatoes with their liquid, the broth,

and 2 cups of water. Bring to a simmer, partially cover, and cook until the cabbage is soft, about 30 minutes.

3. Add the zucchini and bulgur, cover, and cook for 10 minutes. Add the beans and cook 5 minutes longer. Season with additional salt to taste.

Moroccan Vegetable Stew

This aromatic mélange pairs perfectly with couscous or just about any favorite grain. For added color and flavor, sprinkle with freshly chopped mint or parsley before serving. Pass harissa or your favorite hot sauce on the side.

■ 4 TO 6 SERVINGS

2 tablespoons extra virgin olive oil

2 medium red potatoes, coarsely chopped

1 small red bell pepper, diced

3 carrots, peeled and sliced

1 garlic clove, minced

½ teaspoon ground cinnamon

½ teaspoon ground cumin

½ teaspoon ground ginger

1 can (14½ ounces) diced tomatoes, with their juices

¼ cup dried currants or raisins

3 medium zucchini, halved lengthwise and thickly sliced crosswise

1 cup cooked or canned chickpeas, rinsed and drained

1 tablespoon fresh lemon juice

Sea salt and freshly ground pepper

1. In a large flameproof casserole, heat the olive oil over medium heat. Add the potatoes, bell pepper, carrots, garlic, cinnamon, cumin, and ginger. Cook, stirring, until fragrant, about 2 minutes.

2. Add the tomatoes with their juices, 1½ cups water, and the currants.

Bring to a boil. Reduce the heat to medium-low and cook, uncovered, for 15 minutes.

3. Stir in the zucchini, chickpeas, and lemon juice. Cook, partially covered, until the potatoes and zucchini are tender, about 10 minutes. Taste, adding salt and pepper as needed. Serve warm.

12-Minute Ratatouille

Serve this French-style summer vegetable stew as a side dish or as an entree over bulgur, quinoa, or rice. Leftovers make a deliciously different filling for whole wheat pita pockets.

■ 4 TO 6 SERVINGS

    2 tablespoons extra virgin olive oil
    1 medium-large eggplant (about 1 pound), cut into ¾-inch dice
    3 medium zucchini and/or yellow crookneck squash, halved lengthwise
        and cut into ¼-inch-thick slices
    1 small fennel bulb or 2 celery ribs, coarsely chopped
    1 garlic clove, minced
    1 can (14½ ounces) diced tomatoes, with their juices
    ½ teaspoon red wine vinegar
    1 tablespoon chopped fresh thyme or 2 tablespoons chopped fresh
        parsley
    Sea salt and freshly ground pepper

1. In a large flameproof casserole, heat the olive oil over medium heat. Stir in the eggplant, zucchini, fennel, and garlic. Cover and cook for 5 minutes.

2. Stir in the tomatoes with their juices and the vinegar. Partially cover and cook until the vegetables are tender and the juices have thickened slightly, 5 minutes. Stir in the thyme and remove from the heat. Season with salt and pepper to taste. Serve warm, at room temperature, or chilled.

Succotash with Corn, Zucchini, and Green Beans

Colorful and tasty, this vegetable stew can be served over rice as a main dish. It's also good with barley or quinoa. For a lighter meal, pair with Olive Oil–Steamed Spinach (page 252) or steamed chard.

■ 4 SERVINGS

½ pound green beans, trimmed and cut into 1-inch lengths

3 tablespoons minced leek

¾ teaspoon ground cumin

2½ tablespoons extra virgin olive oil

2 cups corn kernels, preferably fresh

1 medium zucchini, halved lengthwise, then sliced

2 large plum tomatoes, coarsely chopped, or half a 14-ounce can diced
    tomatoes

2 tablespoons heavy cream or soy creamer

2 teaspoons fresh lime or lemon juice

Sea salt and crushed hot red pepper

1. Steam the green beans for 3 minutes, or until bright green and tender but still firm.

2. In a large skillet or flameproof casserole, cook the leek with the cumin in the olive oil over medium heat for 2 minutes. Add the corn, raise the heat to medium-high, and sauté, tossing, for 2 minutes longer.

3. Add the zucchini and tomatoes and cook, stirring, for 2 to 3 minutes, until the zucchini begins to soften. Add 1 cup of water and bring to a boil. Partially cover, reduce the heat to medium-low, and simmer, stirring once or twice, until the zucchini is barely tender, about 3 minutes.

4. Add the green beans, heavy cream, and lime juice. Season with salt and hot pepper to taste. Boil over medium-high heat until all the vegetables are tender and the sauce has reduced and thickened slightly.

Zucchini Lasagna

Easy and quick, this tasty vegetable casserole can land on the table in less than half an hour. Serve with a salad or with a side of quinoa or whole wheat pasta, if you like.

■ 3 TO 4 SERVINGS

3 medium zucchini

2 slices whole grain bread

3½ tablespoons extra virgin olive oil

¼ cup lightly packed parsley sprigs

1 tablespoon fresh lemon juice

1 garlic clove, chopped

1 teaspoon dried oregano

Sea salt and freshly ground pepper

¾ cup tomato sauce, preferably homemade

½ cup shredded cheese, preferably half Manchego and half Pecorino
    Romano

1. Preheat the oven to 375°F. Trim the zucchini and cut them lengthwise into ¼-inch slices. Arrange on a rack in a steamer and steam just until barely tender, about 2 minutes. Remove to a plate and let cool slightly.

2. If the bread is moist, toast it very lightly or dry out in a low oven for 10 minutes. Tear the bread into pieces and place in a food processor or blender. Add 2 tablespoons of the olive oil, the parsley, lemon juice, garlic, and oregano. Grind to crumbs. Season with salt and pepper to taste.

3. Generously grease an 8-inch baking or gratin dish with 1½ teaspoons of the olive oil. Arrange a layer of zucchini slices in the bottom of the dish. Sprinkle about one third of the crumbs over the zucchini. Drizzle on ¼ cup of the tomato sauce and sprinkle one third of the cheese over the sauce. Repeat to use up all the ingredients. Drizzle the remaining olive oil over the top.

4. Bake for about 15 minutes, or until the dish is heated through and the top is lightly browned.

Stuffed Giant Zucchini

Here's a delightful vegetarian dish that will serve 6 as a side dish or 4 as a main course, accompanied by a salad. If you can't find a giant zucchini, simply use 2 large.

■ 4 TO 6 SERVINGS

> 1 very large zucchini (about 2½ pounds)
>
> 4½ tablespoons extra virgin olive oil
>
> Sea salt and freshly ground pepper
>
> 1 garlic clove, thinly sliced
>
> ¼ teaspoon crushed hot red pepper
>
> 1 cup coarsely chopped Swiss chard leaves and finely diced stems
>
> 2 medium-small red potatoes, cooked, peeled, and finely diced
>
> 1 cup corn kernels, cooked fresh, thawed frozen, or vacuum packed
>
> ⅓ cup vegetable or chicken broth
>
> 3 tablespoons heavy cream
>
> 1 teaspoon tomato paste
>
> 1 teaspoon black olive tapenade
>
> ¼ cup shredded Pecorino Romano or Manchego cheese

1. Preheat the oven to 350°F. Trim the zucchini and split lengthwise in half. With a large spoon or grapefruit knife, scoop out the pulpy center, leaving a ⅜-inch shell all around. Discard any very seedy parts and finely dice the rest of the scooped-out zucchini. Brush the shells with ½ tablespoon of the oil and bake for 10 to 12 minutes, until they are tender but still hold their shape. Season lightly with salt and pepper and set aside.

2. In a large skillet, heat 3 tablespoons of the olive oil, over medium-high heat. Add the garlic, hot pepper, diced zucchini, and chard stems and sauté for 2 minutes. Add the chopped chard leaves and cook, stirring often, for another 2 minutes. Add the diced potatoes and corn and cook, stirring, until hot, about 2 minutes longer.

3. Stir in the broth, cream, tomato paste, and tapenade. Simmer, stirring often, until most of the liquid is absorbed and the vegetable mixture is thick, 3 to 5 minutes. Remove from the heat and season with salt and pepper to taste.

4. Spoon the vegetable mixture into the zucchini shells, packing it in and mounding it in the center. Sprinkle 2 tablespoons cheese over each half and drizzle with the remaining olive oil. Return to the oven for 5 to 7 minutes, until the dish is hot and the cheese is melted and lightly browned.

BURGERS AND PATTIES

Amaranth Burgers

When amaranth is cooked, it gets sticky, which makes it a good binder. These tasty burgers are served at the Culinarium, the vegetarian luncheon restaurant.

■ 4 SERVINGS

 1 cup whole amaranth

 1 medium-large baking potato (about 8 ounces), peeled and cut into chunks

 1 medium carrot, peeled and sliced

 1 celery rib with leaves, sliced

 3 tablespoons sliced pale green of leek

 2 teaspoons vegetable bouillon powder

 1 teaspoon dried oregano

 Spelt flour

 3 tablespoons extra virgin olive oil

1. Rinse the amaranth well under cold running water. In a small saucepan, cook the amaranth in 2 cups of lightly salted water until it is soft and gluey, 25 to 30 minutes. Transfer to a mixing bowl, cover, and refrigerate until chilled.

2. While the amaranth is cooling, boil the potato in a separate saucepan of salted water until tender, 10 to 15 minutes; drain. When the amaranth is done, add the boiled potato and mash with a fork to a coarse puree. It is fine if some chunks remain.

3. In a food processor, combine the carrot, celery, and leek. Pulse to chop finely. Add to the amaranth and potato along with the bouillon powder and oregano. Mix well. Using the spelt flour on your hands to prevent sticking, form the amaranth mixture into 4 burgers.

4. In a large heavy skillet, heat the olive oil over medium heat. Add the burgers and cook, turning once, until hot throughout and nicely browned on both sides, 3 to 4 minutes per side.

Barley and Black-Eyed Pea Cakes

These substantial cakes will make you forget the meat. Serve with baked sweet potato and an assortment of steamed vegetables, dressed with extra virgin olive oil and freshly squeezed lemon juice.

■ MAKES 8 CAKES; 4 SERVINGS

⅔ cup pearl barley, rinsed

1 can (15 ounces) black-eyed peas, rinsed and drained

⅔ cup whole wheat or spelt bread crumbs

⅓ cup sliced red bell pepper

1 small egg

1 small garlic clove, minced

1 teaspoon dried marjoram

1 teaspoon coarse sea salt

¼ teaspoon freshly ground pepper

¼ cup extra virgin olive oil

1. Bring 2 cups of lightly salted water to a boil in a medium saucepan. Stir in the barley, cover, and reduce the heat to low. Cook the barley until tender but still slightly chewy, 35 to 45 minutes. Uncover, fluff with a fork, and set aside to cool.

2. Place the black-eyed peas, bread crumbs, bell pepper, egg, garlic, and marjoram in a food processor. Pulse 10 times. Season with the salt and pepper.

3. In a large heavy skillet, heat 2 tablespoons of the olive oil. Scoop up ⅓ cup of the black-eyed pea mixture and pack lightly. Place it in the skillet and press lightly with the back of a wide spatula to flatten slightly. Repeat 3 more times to make 4 cakes. Fry, turning once, until nicely browned on the bottom, about 3 minutes. Carefully turn and continue to cook until golden brown and crispy on the second side, about 3 minutes longer. Repeat for a total of 8 cakes.

Black Bean Burgers
with Cashews and Carrots

The marvelous Mark Bittman gave us the idea for combining black beans and oats for a burger that has great texture and looks just like the real thing. These are fine plain, with a squeeze of lemon, or with a big spoonful of Avocado, Corn, and Black Bean Salsa (page 215).

NOTE: If you cook the beans yourself, take them off the heat and drain while they still retain a little texture.

■ MAKES 6 BURGERS; 3 OR 6 SERVINGS

1 large celery rib, coarsely cut up

1 medium-large carrot, peeled and shredded

¼ cup large roasted cashews

2 cups cooked or canned black beans, rinsed and drained well

⅓ cup steel-cut oats

1½ teaspoons vegetable bouillon powder

1 teaspoon ground cumin

1 teaspoon rice vinegar

1 tablespoon extra virgin olive oil, plus more for the pan

Yellow cornmeal

1. Put the celery, carrot, and cashews in a food processor. Pulse to chop coarsely. Add the beans, oats, bouillon powder, cumin, vinegar, and 1 tablespoon olive oil. Pulse until just mixed evenly. Cover and refrigerate for at least 1 hour, or overnight.

2. Form the bean mixture into 6 patties. Dust lightly with cornmeal to coat both sides. Heat the olive oil in a large skillet over medium heat. Add the patties and sauté until lightly browned, 2 to 3 minutes on each side. Or bake in a 375°F oven for about 15 minutes. Let stand for 2 to 3 minutes to firm up before serving.

Lentil and Quinoa Burgers

Because these contain an egg, they hold together better than some moister burgers. Serve with a couple of vegetables or sandwich in a whole wheat pita or whole-grain roll and pair with a nice salad.

■ MAKES 8; 4 SERVINGS

⅔ cup brown lentils, picked over and rinsed

⅔ cup quinoa, rinsed several times

2 tablespoons cornstarch

1 organic egg, lightly beaten

1 tablespoon organic wheat-free tamari

2 teaspoons dried oregano

1 teaspoon ground cumin

¼ teaspoon freshly ground pepper

4 tablespoons extra virgin olive oil

1. Bring 3 cups lightly salted water to a boil in a medium saucepan. Stir in the lentils, partially cover, and cook for 10 minutes. Stir in the quinoa and continue to cook until the lentils are tender but still firm, about 15 minutes longer. Drain and spread out on a baking sheet to cool.

2. Place the cooked lentils and quinoa, cornstarch, egg, tamari, oregano, cumin, and pepper in a food processor and pulse 10 times. Taste and adjust the seasonings if needed.

3. Heat 2 tablespoons of the oil in a large nonstick skillet over medium heat. Scoop up ⅓ cup of the lentil mixture and lightly pack. Place 4 scoops of the mixture into the pan and press lightly with the back of a wide spatula to flatten slightly. Cook the burgers, turning once, until golden brown and crispy on both sides, about 3 minutes per side. Repeat with the remaining oil and lentil mixture. Serve hot.

Curried Vegetable Patties

Potatoes and chickpeas form the base of these substantial patties. Serve with steamed greens and carrots.

■ 6 SERVINGS

4 tablespoons extra virgin olive oil

2 large baking potatoes (10 to 12 ounces each), scrubbed and coarsely grated

¼ cup finely chopped leek (white and pale green)

1½ teaspoons Madras curry powder

¾ cup vegetable stock or water

3 tablespoons fresh lime juice

Sea salt and freshly ground pepper

2 slices (1 ounce each) whole-grain or whole wheat bread, preferably slightly stale, torn into pieces

1½ cups cooked or canned chickpeas, rinsed and drained

¾ cup corn kernels

1. In a large skillet, heat 2 tablespoons of the olive oil over medium–high heat. Add the potatoes, leek, and curry powder. Cook, stirring frequently, for 2 to 3 minutes. Add the vegetable stock and lime juice, reduce the heat to medium, and continue cooking, uncovered, stirring occasionally, until the potatoes are soft and the liquid has been absorbed, about 10 minutes. Season with salt and pepper to taste. Transfer to a large bowl to cool slightly. Do not wash the skillet.

2. If the bread is moist, toast it very lightly. Place the bread in a food processor and pulse to make bread crumbs. (You will have about 1⅓ cups.) Remove and reserve half the crumbs for later. To the crumbs left in the processor, add the chickpeas and corn and process until a coarse puree is formed. Add to the curried vegetables in the bowl, stirring until well blended. Form the mixture into 6 patties, each

about 3 inches across and ¾ inch thick. Gently press the reserved bread crumbs onto both sides of each patty.

3. Heat the remaining oil in the large skillet over medium heat. Add the patties and cook until crisp and golden brown on the outside and heated through, 3 to 4 minutes on a side. Alternatively, arrange the patties 2 inches apart on a lightly greased baking sheet and bake in a 375°F oven for about 20 minutes, turning once, until crisp and golden brown. Serve at once.

CHICKEN, TURKEY, AND FISH

Chicken and Vegetable Curry

Lots of vegetables and a little chicken offer the right balance of nutrition. Serve this flavorful stew over basmati rice.

■ 4 SERVINGS

3 tablespoons extra virgin olive oil

1 inch of fresh ginger, peeled and thinly sliced

1 garlic clove

12 ounces organic, skinless, boneless chicken thighs, cut into 1-inch
   pieces

Sea salt and freshly ground pepper

1½ to 2 tablespoons Madras curry powder

1 can (14 ounces) unsweetened coconut milk

1 cup chicken broth

1½ cups diced cabbage

6 ounces green beans, trimmed and cut into 1-inch lengths

6 organic red new potatoes, scrubbed and quartered

1 tablespoon fresh lemon juice

1. In a spice grinder or mini food processor, puree 2 tablespoons of the olive oil with the ginger and garlic to make a paste. Rub all over the chicken pieces and season with salt and pepper. Let marinate at room temperature for 30 minutes or up to 2 hours in the refrigerator.

2. Heat a large skillet or flameproof casserole over medium heat. Add the chicken with all its marinade and sauté, turning, until the pieces are no longer pink on the outside, 3 to 5 minutes.

3. Sprinkle the curry powder over the chicken and cook, stirring, for 1 to 2 minutes. Pour in the coconut milk and chicken broth. Add the cabbage, green beans, and potatoes and simmer, partially covered, un-

til the vegetables are tender, the chicken is cooked through, and the liquid is slightly thickened, 20 minutes.

4. Stir in the lemon juice and season with additional salt and pepper to taste.

Ginger Chicken Stir-Fry with Carrots, Snow Peas, and Red Pepper

Want dinner on the table in half an hour? Here's a perfect choice. Rice, rice noodles, or even steamed spinach make a fine accompaniment to this easy stir-fry. For extra flavor, you may choose to season the stir-fry with tamari in lieu of additional sea salt before serving.

■ 4 SERVINGS

12 ounces skinless, boneless, organic chicken breasts, trimmed and cut
    into ¾-inch chunks
1 tablespoon minced fresh ginger
Sea salt and freshly ground pepper
2½ tablespoons sunflower oil
1 small red bell pepper, cut into thin strips
2 medium carrots, peeled and thinly sliced
4 ounces fresh snow peas, trimmed
½ cup vegetable or chicken stock
1 tablespoon toasted sesame oil

1. Toss the chicken pieces with 2 teaspoons of the ginger and salt and pepper to taste. Set aside at room temperature for 10 to 15 minutes.

2. In a wok or large heavy skillet, heat 1½ tablespoons of the sunflower oil. Add the chicken pieces and cook for about 2 minutes on each side, until lightly colored outside and no longer pink in the center. Remove the chicken to a bowl. Add the red pepper strips to the wok

and sauté until bright red and barely softened, about 2 minutes. Add to the chicken.

3. Heat the remaining 1 tablespoon sunflower oil in the wok. Add the carrots and remaining 1 teaspoon ginger and cook, tossing, for 2 minutes. Pour in the broth, cover, and cook until the carrots are barely tender, 3 to 4 minutes. Add the snow peas and cook until they are bright green but still crisp, 1 to 2 minutes longer.

4. Return the chicken and red pepper to the wok and cook, tossing with the other vegetables to heat through, 2 to 3 minutes. Season with additional salt and pepper to taste. Drizzle the sesame oil over the stir-fry and serve at once.

Almost Meatless Shepherd's Pie

Barley and corn add nice texture to this savory casserole. For convenience, prepare ahead and bake just before serving.

■ 4 TO 6 SERVINGS

¾ cup pearl barley

½ pound green beans, cut into ½-inch pieces

2 large carrots, peeled and cut into ⅜-inch dice

3 tablespoons extra virgin olive oil

¼ cup thinly sliced leek (white and pale green), well rinsed

½ pound organic turkey breast, cut into ⅜-inch dice

2 tablespoons organic spelt or wheat flour

2 teaspoons organic wheat-free tamari

1 teaspoon thyme leaves, fresh or dried

Sea salt and freshly ground pepper

1 cup corn kernels

Creamy Mashed Potatoes (recipe follows)

1. In a medium saucepan of boiling salted water, cook the barley until it is tender but still pleasantly chewy, 35 to 40 minutes. Drain into a sieve and set aside.

2. While the barley is cooking, steam the green beans and carrots over boiling water until they are just tender, 4 to 5 minutes. Remove from the heat. Measure out and reserve 2 cups of the vegetable broth from the bottom of the steamer.

3. In a large skillet or flameproof casserole, heat 2 tablespoons of the olive oil over medium heat. Add the leek and cook for 1 minute. Add the turkey and continue to cook, stirring occasionally, until the leek is soft and the turkey is no longer pink, about 5 minutes longer.

4. Sprinkle the flour over the turkey and leek and cook, stirring, for 1 minute without browning. Pour in the reserved vegetable broth and bring to a boil, stirring until the liquid is slightly thickened. Add the tamari and thyme. Season generously with salt and pepper. Reduce the heat to medium-low and simmer for 5 minutes. Remove from the heat and let cool slightly. Add the barley, corn, green beans, and carrots. Turn the entire mixture into a 1½-quart casserole, gratin, or shallow baking dish.

5. Preheat the oven to 375°F. Spread the mashed potato topping evenly over the casserole. Swirl decoratively with the back of a spoon. Drizzle the remaining 1 tablespoon olive oil over the top. (The recipe can be prepared to this point several hours or even a day in advance.)

6. Bake the shepherd's pie for 20 to 25 minutes, or until the casserole is piping hot and the potatoes are very lightly browned in spots.

Creamy Mashed Potatoes

■ MAKES ABOUT 3 CUPS

1½ pounds baking potatoes, peeled and cut into 1-inch chunks

2 tablespoons unsalted butter

2 tablespoons heavy cream

¼ teaspoon freshly grated nutmeg

Sea salt and cayenne pepper

1. In a large saucepan of boiling salted water, cook the potatoes until they are tender, 8 to 10 minutes. Scoop out and reserve 1 cup of the cooking water. Drain the potatoes and return them to the pan.

2. Toss the potatoes over low heat until they are dry, 30 to 60 seconds. Remove from the heat and mash with a potato masher or put the potatoes through a ricer or food mill. Beat in the butter, 1 tablespoon at a time, and then the cream.

3. Stir in enough of the reserved cooking water until the mashed potatoes are light and fluffy. Season with the nutmeg and salt and pepper to taste.

Asian-Flavor Cod Baked with Napa Cabbage

Cabbage doubles here as a vegetable and as a wrap to keep the delicate fish moist and tender. Serve with steamed rice or potatoes.

■ 4 SERVINGS

3½ teaspoons extra virgin olive oil

1 head of napa cabbage (about 1 pound)

2 cod fillets, 6 to 8 ounces each

1 teaspoon grated fresh ginger

2 teaspoons organic wheat-free tamari

2 small to medium carrots, cut into matchstick-size pieces or coarsely
  grated

Sea salt

2 teaspoons sesame seeds

1. Preheat the oven to 375°F. Grease a shallow 2-quart baking dish with
   1 teaspoon of the oil. Set aside 4 large outer leaves from the cabbage;
   cut the remaining cabbage crosswise into slices ¼ inch thick and
   spread over the bottom of the baking dish.

2. Cut the cod fillets in half to make 4 equal portions. Spread ¼ teaspoon of the ginger over each fillet; then drizzle with ½ teaspoon of
   the tamari. Divide the carrots equally among the fillets.

3. Cut off the tough stem of each reserved cabbage leaf, so only the
   flexible leafy part remains. Top each fillet with a cabbage leaf and
   wrap, folding in the sides to enclose the fish, as if you were wrapping
   a package. Place seam-side down over the shredded cabbage and drizzle the remaining oil over all. Season lightly with salt and sprinkle the
   sesame seeds on top. Cover tightly with foil and bake for 20 minutes,
   or until the cabbage is tender and the cod is white throughout.

Pecan-Crusted Catfish Fillets

The mildly sweet slaw that follows is a lovely accompaniment to this delicate fish. Accompany also with jasmine or basmati rice.

■ 6 SERVINGS

> ¾ cup pecan halves
>
> ¼ cup yellow cornmeal
>
> ½ teaspoon hot or sweet Hungarian paprika
>
> 1½ tablespoons extra virgin olive oil
>
> Sea salt and freshly ground pepper
>
> 3 skinless catfish fillets, about 6 ounces each
>
> Pineapple Slaw (recipe follows)

1. Preheat the oven to 325°F. Place the pecans on a baking sheet and bake, stirring once or twice, until very lightly browned and fragrant, 5 to 7 minutes. Cool slightly. Increase the oven temperature to 400°F.

2. In a food processor, combine the pecans, cornmeal, paprika, and a dash of salt. Pulse until the pecans are finely chopped. Transfer the mixture to a shallow bowl or plate.

3. Cut the fillets in half and place in a shallow dish. Drizzle with the olive oil and turn to coat. Season with salt and pepper. Dip the fillets in the pecan mixture, pressing gently to coat both sides. Use the oil that remains in the dish to grease a baking sheet; then arrange the fillets without crowding.

4. Bake the catfish for 6 minutes, turn, and then bake for 2 minutes longer, until the fish is golden brown on the outside and opaque throughout. Serve with the slaw on the side.

Pineapple Slaw

■ 4 TO 6 SERVINGS

½ small green cabbage

1 cup pineapple chunks, fresh or unsweetened canned

⅓ cup finely shredded red bell pepper

2 tablespoons rice vinegar

1½ tablespoons sunflower oil

Sea salt and freshly ground pepper

1. Shred the cabbage with a large sharp knife or with the slicing blade of a food processor. Coarsely chop the pineapple.

2. Toss the cabbage with the pineapple, bell pepper, vinegar, and oil. Season with salt and pepper to taste. Let stand at room temperature for at least 30 minutes or refrigerate for 2 hours before serving.

Desserts

While sweets are the least important part of any nutritional program, they are an important part of many people's pleasure. I hope these select recipes, made with lots of fruits, whole grains, and natural sweeteners, will offer the satisfaction and reward so many of us crave. Many of these recipes also can serve as breakfast and between-meal snacks.

Hotel Säntis Amaranth Cake with Bananas
    Vanilla Sauce
Irene's Famous Lemon Tart
Apple Crisp with Pecan Streusel Topping
Maple-Pecan Cookies
Frozen Banana-Maple Mousse
Peachy Mango Mousse
Coconut Tapioca
Maple Baked Apples
Berry Parfait
Glazed Figs with Chestnut Honey and Cashews
Creamy Fruit Salad

Minted Mango and Melon Salad

Apple and Prune Compote

Dried Fruit Compote

Vanilla-Poached Pears with Yogurt Cheese

Poached Plums

Spiced Peaches with Fresh Raspberries

Hotel Säntis Amaranth Cake with Bananas

Popped amaranth is very hard to come by in the United States, but I include this recipe because it is such a favorite with our guests at the Säntis Hotel. If you visit Switzerland, you can buy a package of popped amaranth and bring it back.

■ 8 TO 10 SERVINGS

> 1 package (4 to 5 ounces) popped amaranth
> ¾ cup plus 2 tablespoons white spelt flour
> 1 teaspoon baking powder
> 6 tablespoons unsalted butter
> ½ cup raw brown sugar
> 1 teaspoon vanilla extract
> 2 large ripe but firm bananas, sliced on an angle
> Vanilla Sauce (recipe follows)

1. Preheat the oven to 375°F. Butter a 9 × 5 × 3-inch loaf pan. Line the bottom with parchment or waxed paper and butter the paper.
2. Put the amaranth in a large mixing bowl and set aside. In another bowl, combine the flour with the baking powder. Whisk gently to blend the dry ingredients evenly.
3. Melt the butter and pour into a blender or food processor. Add the brown sugar, vanilla, and 3 tablespoons water. Blend well. Pour the liquid over the amaranth, scraping out the container with a rubber spatula. Mix with a wooden spoon until fluffy. Stir in the dry ingredients just until evenly mixed.
4. Turn half the amaranth batter into the prepared pan. Arrange the banana slices over the batter, filling as many spaces as possible; if there are any banana slices left over, save for garnish. Cover with the remaining batter.

5.   Bake for 22 to 25 minutes, or until the cake begins to pull away from the sides of the pan. Let cool, then cut into small slices and serve with Vanilla Sauce.

Vanilla Sauce
■ MAKES ABOUT 1 CUP

1 cup silken tofu

Seeds from 1 inch of vanilla bean or 1 teaspoon vanilla extract

2 tablespoons maple syrup

Put all the ingredients in a blender or food processor and blend well.

Irene's Famous Lemon Tart
No one will apply the word healthy *to this intensely flavored tart, yet in very small portions the scrumptious dessert is "Dr. Rau approved." It is the creation of Irene Guler, who with her husband Christian runs the Hotel Säntis.*

■ 10 TO 12 SERVINGS

1¾ cups organic white spelt flour

1 stick (4 ounces) cold unsalted butter, cut into tablespoons

Fine sea salt

12 ounces soft silken tofu

1 large organic egg

Juice and zest of 2 lemons

¼ to ⅓ cup mild honey, to taste

1.   Preheat the oven to 400°F.

2.   Add the flour, butter, and a pinch of salt to a food processor. Pulse un-

til the mixture resembles coarse meal. Add about 4 tablespoons ice water and pulse just until the dough begins to come together. If the dough is too crumbly, add 1 more tablespoon ice water. Turn out the dough and press together into a ball. Pat into a flat disc. Wrap and refrigerate for 20 to 30 minutes.

3. On a lightly floured surface, roll out the dough to a thickness of about ¼ inch. Fit the dough into a 9-inch tart pan with a removable bottom, pressing the dough against the sides of the pan. Trim off any extra dough from the top edge of the pan.

4. Bake on the middle rack of the oven for 15 to 18 minutes, or until the pastry is pale golden and set but not browned. Remove from the oven and let cool for 10 minutes. Reduce the oven temperature to 350°F.

5. To make the filling, put the tofu, egg, lemon juice, lemon zest, honey, and a pinch of salt in a blender or food processor. Puree until smooth.

6. Pour the filling into the crust and return to the oven for 12 to 15 minutes, until the filling is just set. Let cool before cutting. Serve at room temperature or chilled.

Apple Crisp with Pecan Streusel Topping

Serve this homey dessert as is or with a drizzle of heavy cream or a dollop of sheep or goat yogurt.

■ 6 SERVINGS

4 tablespoons cold unsalted butter

2¼ pounds sweet-tart apples (about 6), such as Gala or Granny Smith

6 tablespoons raw sugar

Zest and juice of 1 lemon

⅓ cup steel-cut oats

⅓ cup coarsely chopped pecans

¼ cup whole wheat flour

¼ to ½ teaspoon ground cinnamon, to taste

Pinch of sea salt

1. Preheat the oven to 350°F. Lightly grease a 2-quart glass or ceramic baking dish with 1 teaspoon of the butter.

2. Peel and core the apples. Cut them into ½- to ¾-inch wedges and place in the prepared dish. Add 2 tablespoons of the sugar, the lemon juice, and 2 tablespoons of water. Toss gently to mix.

3. In a medium bowl, stir together the remaining ¼ cup sugar, the lemon zest, oats, pecans, flour, cinnamon, and salt. Dice the cold butter and toss with the sugar and nuts. Pinch and rub the mixture between your fingertips until it is the consistency of very coarse meal. Squeeze gently and then release to sprinkle small clumps of the streusel topping evenly over the apples.

4. Bake for 50 minutes, or until the apples are tender and the topping is lightly browned. Serve warm from the oven or at room temperature.

Maple-Pecan Cookies

For some people, spelt is more digestible than other wheats, and it contains more protein and fiber. Most importantly, it is rich in carbohydrates called muco-polysaccharides, which stimulate the immune system. All that aside, these are delicious—and somewhat elegant—cookies.

■ MAKES 2 DOZEN

1 cup spelt flour

1 cup pecan halves

½ teaspoon baking soda

⅛ teaspoon fine sea salt

2 tablespoons unsalted butter, at room temperature

¼ cup maple syrup

1 teaspoon vanilla extract

2 tablespoons sunflower oil

1. Preheat the oven to 350°F. In a food processor, combine the flour, pecans, baking soda, and sea salt. Pulse until the pecans are finely chopped.

2. In a large bowl, beat together the butter and maple syrup with a wooden spoon until light and well blended. Beat in the vanilla, then add the oil in a slow stream, beating well. Add the dry ingredients and stir with the wooden spoon until blended. Drop the dough by rounded teaspoons onto a buttered cookie sheet.

3. Bake for 12 minutes, or until the cookies are just beginning to brown around the edges. Transfer to a wire rack and let cool before eating.

Frozen Banana-Maple Mousse

Yogurt can transform just about any ripe fruit into a refreshing frozen mousse. A topping of toasted macadamia nuts provides a contrasting crunch that complements the subtle maple flavor.

■ 4 SERVINGS

2 ripe bananas, cut into chunks

2 to 3 tablespoons pure maple syrup

1 cup unflavored goat or sheep yogurt

2 tablespoons toasted chopped macadamia nuts, for garnish

1. Combine the bananas and maple syrup in a blender or food processor. Process, pulsing the machine on and off, until a coarse puree forms. Add the yogurt, pulsing just until blended.

2. Scrape the mixture into 4 ramekins or parfait glasses. Cover with plastic wrap and freeze for at least 1 hour, or until firm.

3. Just before serving, top each with 1 tablespoon of toasted macadamia nuts. This is best served the same day it is made.

Peachy Mango Mousse

Mangoes are rich in vitamins, minerals, digestive enzymes, and fiber. More importantly for dessert, they taste delicious.

■ 4 SERVINGS

2 large ripe mangoes (14 to 15 ounces each), peeled

¼ cup silken tofu

1 cup peach nectar

1 envelope (¼ ounce) unflavored gelatin

1. Peel the mangoes and cut the fruit away from the pit, cutting as close to the seed as possible. Puree the mango in a food processor or blender until smooth. (There will be about 1½ cups.)
2. Add the tofu and process until smooth. Scrape the mixture into a large bowl.
3. Pour the peach nectar into a small saucepan and stir in the gelatin. Let stand for 5 to 10 minutes, until softened. Cook over low heat just until the gelatin dissolves and the mixture is heated through.
4. Gradually whisk the peach nectar into the mango puree. Pour the mixture into a serving bowl or 4 dessert dishes or parfait glasses. Cover and refrigerate until set, about 2 hours.

Coconut Tapioca
■ 4 SERVINGS

¼ cup instant tapioca
1 can (14 ounces) coconut milk
⅓ cup maple syrup
2 teaspoons vanilla extract

1. In a nonreactive medium saucepan, combine the tapioca, coconut milk, maple syrup, and 1 cup of water. Stir well. Let stand for 5 minutes.
2. Bring the mixture to a boil over medium-low heat, stirring frequently. Remove from the heat, stir in the vanilla, and let cool slightly. To prevent a skin from forming on the top of the tapioca, place a sheet of plastic wrap directly on the surface of the pudding. Serve at room temperature or chill in the refrigerator to serve cold.

Maple Baked Apples

■ 4 SERVINGS

4 large baking apples, such as Cortland or Granny Smith

1½ teaspoons fresh lemon juice

¼ cup raisins

¼ cup chopped pecans

1 teaspoon ground cinnamon

¼ cup maple syrup

4 teaspoons butter, at room temperature

1. Preheat the oven to 350°F. Core the apples, being careful to leave the bottom intact. With a vegetable peeler, peel a 1-inch strip from around the outside of the top core. Sprinkle the lemon juice into the apples to prevent browning.

2. In a small bowl, mix the raisins, pecans, and cinnamon. Stuff the raisin-pecan mixture into each apple. Drizzle 1 tablespoon of maple syrup into each. Top with the remaining filling, mounding any extra on top. Dot each apple with 1 teaspoon butter.

3. Place the apples in a small baking dish and pour 1 cup of water into the bottom of the pan. Put the pan in the middle of the oven and bake for 30 minutes, or until the apples are just tender.

Berry Parfait

Whether you make this with fresh berries in summer or with frozen in winter, it's a lovely dessert no one will think of as health food. Tip: Don't tell anyone it's goat yogurt, and no one will guess.

■ 4 SERVINGS

2 cups fresh or frozen strawberries

1¼ cups fresh or frozen raspberries

1 cup fresh or frozen blueberries

1 container (8 ounces) plain goat yogurt, such as Redwood Hill Farms

2 tablespoons raw brown sugar

2 tablespoons unsweetened shredded coconut or chopped pecans

1. Rinse the berries. Hull the strawberries and remove any stems from the blueberries.
2. In a blender or food processor, combine the yogurt, brown sugar, 1 cup of the strawberries, and ½ cup of the raspberries. Puree until smooth.
3. Slice or quarter the remaining strawberries. Toss them with the remaining raspberries and the blueberries. In 4 tall parfait glasses, wine-glasses, or glass dessert dishes, layer the berries and berry yogurt alternately. Sprinkle the coconut or pecans on top.

Glazed Figs with Chestnut Honey and Cashews

These lovely fresh figs make a nice morning snack, or they can be combined with Yogurt Cheese (page 296) or a nice fresh goat cheese for a lovely dessert.

■ 4 SERVINGS

4 fresh figs, black or green

4 teaspoons chestnut honey

3 tablespoons chopped cashews

1. Preheat the broiler. Slice the figs from top to bottom, leaving them just slightly attached at the base. Fan them out to open up the slices as much as possible and arrange on a lightly oiled baking sheet. Drizzle 1 teaspoon of the honey over each fig.

2. Broil about 4 inches from the heat for 2 minutes, or until the honey is just melted and the figs are hot. Watch carefully so they don't burn.

3. Serve warm or at room temperature, with chopped cashews sprinkled on top.

Creamy Fruit Salad

As always, be sure to choose organic fruit. Not only is it more nutritious, you will find it is fresher and tastes much better than ordinary produce.

■ 4 SERVINGS

> 1 large green apple, cut into ½-inch chunks
>
> 1 banana, sliced
>
> 1 teaspoon fresh lemon juice
>
> 24 seedless red grapes, halved if large
>
> 2 to 3 teaspoons honey
>
> ¼ teaspoon ground cinnamon
>
> 1 cup plain goat yogurt

1. Toss the apple and banana with the lemon juice to prevent discoloration. Add the grapes.
2. Stir 2 teaspoons of the honey and the cinnamon into the yogurt until well blended. Add the third teaspoon honey if you think it needs it, keeping in mind the fruit is sweet.
3. Add the sweetened yogurt to the fruit and fold gently to mix.

Minted Mango and Melon Salad

You can enjoy this refreshing fruit salad at breakfast, as a midmorning snack, or as dessert at lunch. If you have any fresh strawberries or blueberries in the house, they would make a very nice addition. Remember, to avoid fermentation of undigested fruit overnight, it is highly recommended you eat no raw fruit after 4:00 in the afternoon. At night, choose one of the poached fruit compotes or another cooked dessert.

NOTE: When mangoes are ripe, they feel like firm ripe peaches.

■ 4 SERVINGS

> 2 mangoes
>
> 2 cups diced melon (honeydew, cantaloupe, and/or watermelon)
>
> 2 teaspoons honey
>
> ¼ cup freshly squeezed orange juice
>
> 2 teaspoons slivered fresh mint leaves

1. Peel the mangoes, cut the fruit off the pit, and dice it. *Or* cut the unpeeled fruit off the wide flat pit, which makes the mango easier to handle. Then score the fruit into cubes without cutting through the skin. Bend the skin backward and the fruit will either come right off or can be coaxed off the skin easily with a small knife.
2. Place the diced mango and the melon in a pretty serving bowl.
3. In a small bowl, dissolve the honey in the orange juice. Pour over the fruit, add 1 teaspoon of the mint, and toss to mix. Let macerate at room temperature for 15 to 30 minutes, stirring occasionally. Serve garnished with the remaining mint.

Apple and Prune Compote

This can be eaten for breakfast or dessert. Serve with a small drizzle of heavy cream or a dollop of plain goat yogurt, if you like.

■ 6 SERVINGS

2 large apples, peeled, cored, and thinly sliced

1 cup pitted prunes

1 wide strip of lemon zest, about 2 inches long

1 cinnamon stick

2 teaspoons honey

1. Place all the ingredients in a medium saucepan with 2 cups of water. Bring to a boil, reduce the heat to low, and cover. Simmer the compote for 10 minutes.
2. Remove from the heat and let stand, covered, until cool. Serve warm, at room temperature, or slightly chilled.

Dried Fruit Compote

When fresh fruit choices diminish during the winter months, organic dried fruits, which contain no sulfur, are a welcome substitute. Since they are so concentrated, they are naturally sweet and require no additional sugar or honey. Leave the larger fruits whole, if you like, or cut them into bite-size pieces.

NOTE: Be sure all the dried fruits you buy are organic and sulfur-free.

■ 6 SERVINGS

1 cup dried apricots

1 cup dried pears

1 cup dried apples

¾ cup dried figs, stems removed, halved if large

1 teaspoon grated zest and juice from 1 lemon

1 cinnamon stick, broken in half

1 tablespoon finely diced crystallized ginger

1. Combine all the ingredients in a nonreactive medium saucepan. Add
    1½ cups water and bring to a boil. Reduce the heat to low and sim-
    mer slowly for 10 minutes, stirring occasionally.

2. Remove from the heat, cover, and let the fruits cool to room temper-
    ature in the syrup. Serve the compote at room temperature or slightly
    chilled.

Vanilla-Poached Pears with Yogurt Cheese

Poached pears are a light and lovely dessert that can follow just about any meal.
For best flavor, choose Bartletts; for best texture, Bosc or Anjou.

■ 4 SERVINGS

4 ripe but firm pears

1 cup unsweetened apple juice

½ lemon

1 piece of vanilla bean (about 2 inches), split lengthwise in half

1 cinnamon stick, broken into 2 or 3 pieces

Yogurt Cheese (recipe follows)

1. Peel the pears. Use a long apple corer to remove the cores from the
    bottom, leaving just the stems intact.

2. In a large wide saucepan or flameproof casserole, combine the apple
    juice with ⅔ cup water. Cut several strips of zest from the lemon
    half, making sure to avoid the white pith. Squeeze the juice into the
    pot. With the tip of a small knife, scrape the tiny seeds from the
    vanilla bean into the liquid; toss in the pod, as well. Add the cinna-
    mon stick.

3.   Bring the poaching liquid to a simmer over medium-low heat. Arrange the pears on their sides in the pan. Don't worry if they are not completely covered with liquid. Partially cover the pot and simmer, rolling the pears gently to turn them several times, until they are just tender, 15 to 20 minutes.

4.   With a slotted spoon, remove the pears and let cool. Boil the syrup in the pan until reduced by about a third and flavorful. Chill, if desired. Serve each pear with a few tablespoons of syrup and a dollop of Yogurt Cheese on top.

Yogurt Cheese

This simple thickened yogurt is easy to make and amazingly versatile. It can be mixed with herbs and served as a savory spread or used plain or sweetened as a topping for desserts.

▦ MAKES ABOUT 1 CUP

2 cups (1 pint) plain goat or sheep yogurt

1.   Line a fine sieve with a double thickness of damp cheesecloth. Place the sieve over a deep bowl to catch the whey. (Be sure the sieve does not touch the bottom of the bowl.)

2.   Without stirring, gently spoon the yogurt into the sieve and let drain, covered, in the refrigerator until thickened but still soft, 24 to 48 hours. Drain the whey. If made in advance, cover and refrigerate the yogurt cheese for up to 1 week.

Poached Plums

Only mildly sweetened with natural juice, this is a good fruit to have with porridge in the morning, along with some of the poaching liquid to moisten the cereal.

■ 4 SERVINGS

> 5 ripe purple plums or 10 prune plums
>
> 1 cup pear nectar

1. Rinse the plums well and dry. With a small sharp knife, cut the plums in half. Remove the pits.
2. Place the plum halves and pear nectar in a medium saucepan. Add additional water, if needed, to cover. Bring to a simmer and cook just until the plums soften, about 5 minutes.
3. Serve warm, at room temperature, or slightly chilled.

Spiced Peaches with Fresh Raspberries

A bowl of these lovely peaches and a couple of Maple-Pecan Cookies (page 286) would make a dessert fit for company. When peaches are out of season, plums or even pears can be cooked in similar fashion; neither of these fruits need peeling.

■ 4 SERVINGS

> 1 pound ripe peaches
>
> ¼ cup unsweetened 100% fruit jam, such as raspberry, strawberry, or
>   apricot
>
> Grated zest and juice of 1 lemon
>
> ¼ teaspoon ground cinnamon
>
> 1 cup raspberries

1. Bring a large pot of water to a boil. Add the peaches and blanch for 10 to 15 seconds to loosen the skins. Drain and rinse under cold running water. The skins should slip right off.

2. Halve the peaches and remove the pits. Cut each half into 4 or 5 wedges.

3. In a nonreactive medium saucepan, combine the fruit jam, lemon zest, lemon juice, cinnamon, and ¾ cup water. Bring to a boil over medium heat, stirring to mix. Reduce the heat to a simmer. Add the peaches and poach until just tender, 7 to 10 minutes.

4. Immediately remove from the heat and let cool to room temperature, about 1 hour. Then add the raspberries. Serve at once or refrigerate in the syrup for up to 4 days in an airtight container. Be sure to include a few tablespoons of the poaching liquid in each dish. Save the rest of the poaching liquid to use on porridge.

Exploring the Swiss Biological Medicine Network

Now that you have a better understanding of what Swiss biological medicine is all about, you may want to take it a step further. In your own home you can practice the basic nutrition, which is extremely important. But if you have a medical problem or symptoms that have not been diagnosed, you may want to pursue more targeted treatment.

Of course, I hope you will come to see me in Switzerland at our Paracelsus Clinic. And twice a year, we offer cleansing weeks, with lectures in English, at Al Ronc. But there are also many practitioners throughout the United States who have studied with me and who have much to offer. Some of them provide follow-up.

The problem with simply listing these clinics and individual practitioners is that they vary so widely. Some have comprehensive clinics and are excellent for overall care or for follow-up treatments after a visit to Paracelsus. Others offer discrete specialized services, such as holistic dentistry, homeopathy, acupuncture, herbal treatments, Chinese medicine, and massage therapy. Because deciding what you need and who to see can be confusing to any patient, especially one new to Swiss biological medicine, we have established the Paracelsus Biological Medicine Network. This nonprofit organization operates out of Marion, Massachusetts. The full-time staff there is dedicated to screening patients over the phone and through detailed questionnaires so that they can direct them appropriately to me or direct them to other biological medicine doctors and treatments.

Contact the Paracelsus Biological Medicine Network by calling 508-748-0816. Write to the Paracelsus Biological Medicine Network, c/o The Marion Institute, 3 Barnabas Road, Marion, MA 02738. Or go to the website at www.pbmn.org. Contact the clinic directly by e-mail at www.paracelsus.ch, or go directly to my website at DrRau.com.

Sources for Organic Foods

Organic fruits and vegetables, poultry, eggs, dairy, and grocery items as well as nutritional supplements have long been available in health food shops and in natural and organic markets like Wild Oats. Because of the many health benefits of organic foods, as well as their superior taste and quality, upscale supermarkets such as Wegman's, Fairway, and Whole Foods now carry fresh organic produce. They also devote entire aisles to high-quality organic groceries, baked goods, cereals, goat yogurt, and flax seed oil, as well as bulk grains, beans, and rice, among other items you'll need to follow Dr. Rau's Way. And now that the USDA has given legal significance to the term "certified organic," many other stores, such as Wal-Mart, are offering wider and broader selections of organics.

In summer, look for local organic growers near where you live. Many sell their produce at farmers' markets, which are burgeoning all over the country. Community Supported Agriculture (CSA) programs are growing as well; these charge an annual fee, which supports the farmer, and you receive a basket of whatever is ripe every week throughout the season.

What you lose in choice you gain in quality. Also, keep an eye out for local free-range organic poultry.

In winter, or if you prefer to shop over the Internet for convenience, there are many online sources for excellent organic produce and grocery items, which deliver overnight. Some offer convenient plans you can set up so you automatically receive a basket of fresh organic produce every week or once a month. Perishables are shipped overnight via UPS or FedEx. Often there is no extra shipping charge, but, of course, the cost is built into the price of your order. Nonetheless, especially in winter, they make it possible to eat well without having to leave your home. Here is a sampling:

Door to Door Organics

Devoted exclusively to fresh organic fruits, vegetables, and herbs, this is an excellent company with an easy-to-use website and excellent customer service. You can order once or sign up for a regular box. There is choice of frequency as well as size and composition of order. Every week, you're sent e-mail notification that your order has been placed. You go to the website to see what is in that week's box. You may substitute items if you wish. You can also custom order other fruits and vegetables. (www.doorto doororganics.com / 888-283-4443)

ShopNatural

First established as a local co-op in Tucson, Arizona, in 1974, the not-for-profit organization now serves the entire country through its website. Its online grocery store is well stocked with a wide range of nonperishable foods as well as supplements and other home items. Its products are thoroughly vetted and well priced, especially if you buy in bulk. (www.shop natural.coop / 800-350-2667)

Diamond Organics

Since they're located on the Monterey Peninsula in California, and most of the organic produce is locally grown, you know the quality of this produce is special. But it's got a price tag to match. Best values are the samplers. If you don't see one online that matches your needs, customer service can help you put together a personalized order. (www.diamond organics.com / 888-674-2642)

If you're enterprising, the most economical way to eat organic foods is by setting up your own food co-op with a few like-minded friends. This can be done with local farmers, or through **United Natural Foods, Inc.**, the largest—and oldest—food co-op in the country. Their grocery division—canned goods, bulk beans, grains, rice, flour, etc.—has ten distribution centers throughout the United States. Their fresh produce division, **Albert's Organics**, which also sells some natural meats and poultry, has six. If you are anywhere near one of their routes, a minimum order of $250 will cost only $7.50 extra for delivery. Customer service at the number below will direct you to the distribution center closest to your location. (www.unfi.com / 800-451-2525; www.albertsorganics.com / 888-289-8418)

INDEX